INSIGHT into LOW VISION

Terri Cyr, OD

Vision Insight Publications

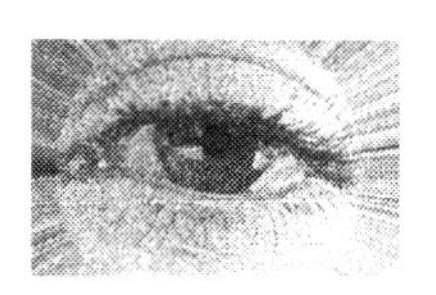

ISBN: 978-0-9972453-0-1

Library of Congress Control Number: 2016901272

Edited by: Rebecca Ann Meyer

Cover and book design by: Patricia Rasch (bookandcoverdesign.com)

insightintolowvision.com

Vision Insight Publications

Connecticut, USA

DEDICATION

David, Joe, and Christine for their love and understanding.

ACKNOWLEDGEMENT

Thank you to my business associate, Linda Caliolo, OD, for having confidence in me when I had lost confidence in myself.

About this Book

The intention of the author in writing this book was to bring together information which is helpful to those with subnormal vision. This book is a reference guide and starting point for those who desire to know more about resources and technologies available to those with vision loss. All the information is accurate to the author's best knowledge, and up-to-date at the time of writing. While this guide is a helpful source of information, it is not intended to take the place of those knowledge professionals who work with the visually impaired.

The author chose to format this book in large print, with adequate line spacing, and bold print to make it more accessible for those with subnormal vision.

Contents

CHAPTER 11

CHAPTER 12

CHAPTER 13

Introduction

I hate eye exams. I would rather go to the dentist than have an eye exam. Peculiar, since I am an eye doctor, that is, an optometrist by trade.

My aversion to eye exams started when I received the bad news. I worked as an optometrist for 18 years. I have seen the dejected look in the eyes of my patients. Those eyes that could no longer see as well, but could express the quiet despair of loss.

Even if they came into my office with some anticipation of me giving them hope, I had to deliver the bad news. My verdict was usually that their vision was 'a little worse.' Vision would never get any better for these patients. They knew this on a subconscious level before they came in for their eye exam, but now their hope was gone.

I admit I am not any different from my patients. There were subtle changes in vision. Changes that on a daily basis I adapted to and chose to ignore. Not me! I chalked it up to getting older. It, I assured myself, is normal.

So now here I am in a retina specialist's office, but I know too much, there is no hope here. Mine is a degenerative eye disease. I could not ignore it any longer. It was my turn to sit in the chair opposite to where I was used to sitting. This time the bad news was for me. All the suspicions I had about how my patients felt when they got the bad news, washed over me like the proverbial tsunami. I knew it was coming, but could never be totally prepared. I remember saying casually "Yeah, I suspected that. I am an optometrist you know!" Then I sat as cooperative as I could, maintaining my composure, through the barrage of tests that followed. I also learned that you have to drive home carefully when your mind is consumed with your personal grief and your eyes are filled with tears. This particular driving skill comes in handy as it is the ritual every time I go for an eye exam.

Years ago, when my vision was a perfect 20/20 with no eyeglass correction, I remember something I had said while sitting with a group of optometrists and ophthalmologists over dinner. The conversation turned to the practice of Low Vision. The doctors were discussing the satisfaction of helping people who were losing their vision and giving them hope. "I don't agree" I said. "I find it depressing, and insurance doesn't pay." I have learned a lot since those days.

There was the grief and sadness, combined with the bouts of despair and denial. I moved backward, before I moved forward, until I finally came to terms with the realization that my life was not over. I wrote this book to bring together the knowledge I have as an optometrist, and the information I think will be helpful to others. I don't know if this gives hope, but I believe that knowledge is power.

Oh…and insurance still doesn't pay.

Terri Cyr, OD

CHAPTER 1

A Chapter for Family and Friends

Dear Family and Friends,

Forget all your preconceived notions of blindness and vision loss. Each person has a different story. There are different degrees of vision loss, just as there are different degrees to which an individual accepts and adjusts to their loss.

Grief and sadness are normal. Vision loss is losing a part of yourself. The freedom, control, and power I felt as an independent seeing person was slipping away. It is like the loss you feel for a loved one. "How can I go on? Will I be totally blind one day?" This is my fear. Things that used to be so easy are now a struggle. Everything takes more time and effort. Sometimes I wonder if it is all worthwhile.

I may be losing my vision, but I have not lost my mind. My senses of hearing and touch are not really any better; I am just paying more attention now.

Sometimes I feel alone in a crowd. There is a sense I am not like the others. I feel conspicuous in my attempt to appear normal. I cannot recognize faces like I used to do, never mind interpreting facial expressions or reading into someone's eyes. I miss those nuances of social interaction.

Out in public, people do not understand. They look at you queerly, or get impatient if your interaction with them is not quick enough or to their satisfaction. I hesitate to launch into the litany about how I can't see very well for fear of drawing sympathetic remarks or unwanted attention to myself.

You do not realize how important reading is until you lose your capability to see the fine detail reading requires. This means a loss of sources of information and communication. Packaging labels, newspapers, photographs, clocks, computers, signs, and even television have printed material which has become difficult to read.

Often I may feel frustrated because I cannot see what others are seeing, such as signs, stages, and other distant points of interest. (By the way, I hate movies that randomly insert subtitles.) Worst of all, I am frustrated that my job, hobbies, and activities have all changed. Each time I am faced with something I can no longer do, it is a reminder of my losses. I might hide it well, but I am sad.

I need your help. But please remember, there is a fine line between helping me help myself, and doing it for me, leaving me with a feeling of helplessness and dependency. Sometimes, because everything seems so much more difficult, I just wish you would take care of it all for me. But down deep, for my own psychological well-being, I know I must create my new independence.

My best option is to get the help of qualified professionals. These are usually optometrists or ophthalmologists, and rehabilitation specialists, who will evaluate where I am in terms of my disabilities, needs, and desires for daily life functioning. These evaluations are for problem solving. I know that there is not one magical vision aid, but the low vision specialist has the knowledge and access to a wide range of options, depending on my needs. This includes not just the magnifiers that we see in department stores, but a large spectrum of specialized glasses, magnifiers, telescopes, and technologies. These things can help open those closed doors and reconnect me to my world.

The low vision specialist can also help me get access to rehabilitative services. This does not mean they will help get my vision back, but it does mean they can help me learn to use what vision I have left. It also includes mobility training and school, work, and household adaptive techniques. This is all about learning new skills. The specialist is usually familiar with other agencies that can help.

Finally, if I am not making any progress and I seem disinterested, incommunicative, and reclusive, I may be suffering with depression and anxiety. Whereas grief and sadness are normal with the onset of vision loss, long-term depression, although common, is not normal. I may need the help of a psychiatric evaluation and/or a support group. It is good to know that there are others out there struggling as I do.

Most of all I need for you to be supportive, understanding and patient. I don't need sympathy and pity. I am a capable and competent person. I do not live in darkness, but it is a new world for me and I must learn, with your help and the knowledge of professionals, to embrace it, and keep moving forward.

Sincerely,

Be not afraid of going slowly,
Be afraid only of standing still.
Chinese Proverb

CHAPTER 2

Impairment, Disability, or Handicap?

The World Health Organization defined these three terms: 'An **impairment** is any loss or abnormality of psychological, physiological, or anatomical structure or function; a **disability** is any restriction or lack (resulting from an impairment) of ability to perform an activity in the manner or within the range considered normal for a human being; a **handicap** is a disadvantage for a given individual, resulting from an impairment or a disability, that prevents the fulfillment of a role that is considered normal (depending on age, sex and social and cultural factors) for that individual'. (1)

Impairment is the physical aspect and disability are constraints and restrictions because of the impairment. Loss of vision is your impairment. The visual system is somehow damaged or altered, and is not functioning as well as eyes of 'normal' people. Disability is the disadvantage you must work through to integrate yourself into your community and prevent yourself from becoming isolated.

We live in a sighted world, in which the norm has been established as a 20/20 (6/6) visual acuity (or better). Contemporary life is based on this standard. So much of our society revolves around the printed word. The capability to read the printed word is the key to accessibility (transportation, activities, and leisure sports), general communication (signs and computers), and personal interaction (cell phones and messaging). The inability of those with vision loss to see and therefore benefit from the printed word is the disability.

It is the combination of your capabilities for adjustment and adaption, along with the support of friends, family, and the community that will help you maintain a life of normalcy.

Handicaps should be left to the game of golf. A handicap is given to the less skilled and less capable player. It is like getting a hand-out, instead of a hand-up, and is tied to a social perception of that person as not being up to par. It defines the disabled individual's place in society as being 'less than' or less competent.

The term handicapped has fallen into social disfavor. (I laugh thinking about the 1990's term '**handi**-capable'.) I suspect that is why it is called the Americans with Disabilities Act, and not the American with Handicaps Act. The Americans with Disabilities Act is all about assimilating those with disabilities into society, and removing restrictions and constraints that set them apart, because they are not 'normal' by social standards. Perhaps our collective social conscience is that we are all grown up now and we feel that we have done what we can do to accept and give access to those with disabilities. So with the combination of the social movement toward accessibility, contemporary innovations, and leaps in technology, ask yourself: Am I disabled or am I handicapped? Will

I define myself by my poor vision, or do I have other capabilities that can help me move beyond my impairment?

Our social history is marked by the lives of individuals, who despite their visual impairment, went on to productive lives. Claude Monet continued painting for many years after cataracts took away his fine vision. He adapted by painting the large water lily sequence. (2) Harriet Tubman, known for her courageous work with the Underground Railroad to free slaves, had herself lost vision when she took a blow to the head while working as a slave. (3) Andre Bocelli is a profoundly popular and inspirational classical singer, who lost his vision as a 12 year old boy. He once played piano and soccer, but then turned his focus to singing. (4) Marla Runyan (5), Brian McKeever, and Erik Weihemayer are all visually impaired and are premier world-class athletes. There are many who learn to redefine their job skills and go on to have successful careers. There are visually disabled who are teachers, nurses, computer technicians, and even librarians. Social attitudes and technology have opened the door of accessibility to the visually impaired, who are willing to challenge the 'norm' and hopefully make ' handicap' a thing of the past.

Blind, Legally Blind, and Low Vision

The general social view of blindness is that there is an inability to see and that darkness prevails. But that is not always the case. The American Medical Association first established a definition of blindness that was taken up by the Social Security Administration, to set eligibility guidelines (6), and by the judicial system as a legal definition .

'**Legal blindness**' is defined as visual acuity no better than 20/200 (6/60) in the better eye with best prescription for eyeglasses or contact lenses. The top number represents how many feet (or meters) away the target letter is located. The bottom number is less easy to describe, as it is a measurement based on degrees and minutes of arc with some trigonometry thrown in. Simply said, at 20 feet (6 meters), the 20/20 (6/6) letter is 8.75 mm in height or about a 3/8 of an inch. Therefore, the individual with 20/200 (6/60) vision can see a letter only if it is 87.5 mm or 3 5/8 inches tall at 20 feet (6 meters). Another way to say it is that someone with 20/200 (6/60) vision can see at only 20 feet (6 meters) what others with normal vision can see at 200 feet (60 meters), wearing their best set of eyeglasses or contact lenses. Both eyes can be the same, or one eye can be worse, but the better eye can only see 20/200 (6/60) for the legal blindness status.

Legal blindness is also defined in terms of visual field. The definition is that a central viewing area with a diameter of 20 degrees or less is considered legally blind. Compare that to fully sighted individual with a horizontal visual field of 180 to 190 degrees. It is possible for the visual acuity in the small central area to be a normal 20/20, but there is no peripheral vision. Legally blind visual field loss is like viewing life through a keyhole.

Those in either of the two categories of legally blind, although they experience a vision disability, can still have usable vision remaining. Keep in mind 'legally blind' parameters are used as guidelines by social and government agencies. These agencies do best with lines and numbers. If their vision is better than 20/200 or their visual field is larger than 20 degrees, the low vision patient is disqualified from receiving the 'legally blind' title, and cannot take advantage of some state and federal benefits and services. These numbers, however, do not give any insight into what functional vision remains and how the individual functions with that residual vision. The reality is that legally blind, in most cases, is not blind at all by a true dictionary type definition:

Blind (adj) without the power of sight, unable to see, sightless.
(Webster's New World Dictionary, 1968. The only dictionary I have, I use the internet dictionary now)

Most of the legally blind are actually best described as having low vision. What defines low vision? Low vision is defined as visual acuity no better than 20/70 (6/21) in the better eye, but better than the legally blind defined limit of 20/200 (6/60). Again, this is with the best eyeglass or contact lens prescription in the better eye for the person being measured. The low vision group will also include those with varying degrees of visual field loss and blind spots (scotomas), which can also hinder visual function.

There is a wide spectrum of people with low vision, ranging from mild to severe functional vision losses. You can attach some numbers to these losses, like visual acuity, visual field losses, or loss of contrast sensitivity, but how the individual functions can vary widely from person to person. Factors such as age, age of impairment onset, general health, psychological well-being, stability of the vision loss process, social and family support, and receipt of eye care and rehabilitative services, will influence how an individual functions with their vision loss. (7)

The takeaway message here is that many 'legally blind' are low vision (visually impaired, partially sighted, visually challenged, visually disabled, pick one), but not all who have low vision are legally blind.

References

1. World Health Organization. Document A29/INFDOCI/1, Geneva, Switzerland, 1976.
2. Crespella, Jean-Paul. Monet The Masterworks. New York, Portland House, 1096, pg 136.
3. Famous People With Vision Impairments Past and Present. Disabled World. (2015) Retrieved from **www.disabled-world.com/artman/publish/famous-blind.shtml**.
4. Andrea Bocelli. (2015). The **Biography.com** website. 07:25, Retrieved Jul 30, 2015, from **http://www.biography.com/people/andrea-bocelli-9216943**.
5. *About*. (2015) Retrieved from **www.marlarunyan.net**.
6. Social Security Administration, Federal Register, (71 FR 67037) 2006.
7. Brown, Barbara. The Low Vision Handbook for Eyecare Professionals, 2nd Ed., SLACK incorporated, 2007.

CHAPTER 3

Acceptance – Adjustment - Adaption

The Serenity Prayer

God grant me the serenity
to accept the things I cannot change;
courage to change the things I can;
and wisdom to know the difference.

Living one day at a time;
Enjoying one moment at a time;
Accepting hardships as the pathway to peace;
Taking, as He did, this sinful world
as it is, not as I would have it;
Trusting that He will make all things right
if I surrender to His Will;
That I may be reasonably happy in this life
and supremely happy with Him
Forever in the next.
Amen.

—Reinhold Niebuhr

ACCEPTANCE

Some things will never be the same.

Acceptance is the most difficult step. You can't move forward without accepting what has come to be. The rest will follow.

Each time I noticed a change in my vision, my first reaction was of despair, accompanied by a flood of tears. Even now, I can't think about those milestones without a sense of sadness. Looking back, I can still feel the pain of those moments. My life was changing and even with all my knowledge, I was powerless to stop it. Each change disabled me from another activity. There was a lot of looking forward, thinking about my future, and mourning what was not to be. Not only was I sad, but I was also fearful. I had created an identity for myself: "I am well educated, efficient, capable, and a multi-tasker." I was afraid of losing myself.

Initially there was the denial. Mine was that there was only a little vision change, "Certainly it won't get any worse. I will do all the right things, it will remain stable, and I'll be fine. I can deal with this." Then denial would smack me in the head by the reality of more vision loss. The cycle of denial, then the reality breakdown, would repeat itself until I could deny it no longer. My vision loss had changed my life. I had worked hard to get to where I was in my profession, and I did not want to give it up. I was sad for how things would have been different without this burden of vision loss. I felt the degeneration, not only of my vision, but of my life.

My depression waxed as my self-esteem crumbled. Our perception of ourselves is influenced by the people around us.

My fear was that I would be viewed by others as being 'less than' or 'incapable'. I had a sense of not being useful to either myself or those around me, and I did not have the power, so I thought, to do anything about it.

Depression is normal. It is that unrelenting sadness that hangs over you. It is not proportional to the severity of the disability. The degree to which it affects each of us is different. Some (like me) will deny their depression. Others become consumed. It causes lack of interest and lack of motivation. Seeing less can lead to doing less, and the result is a feeling of isolation. Fear and anxiety arise from the sense of helplessness. Anger can arise from these frustrations and alienate those who are most important to us, and even destroy relationships. The visually impaired rarely report their depression to eye care professionals, family, and friends.

All these emotions of denial, anger, fear, anxiety, and depression, although not unexpected, are counterproductive to our acceptance.

I permitted myself to mourn each perceptible loss. Grieving is an important step. Even now a little sadness and envy rises up in me when I notice others can see what I can't see. I cry, mostly from frustration, only rarely now. Understanding that some things will never be the same is acceptance.

ADJUSTMENT

One day at a time.

My acceptance was not over night. After each good crying session, I pulled myself together with a little more resolve to move on. I thought too much of myself to let this overtake me and drag me down. A new normal would have to be established. For every individual the process is different. The process is difficult to do on your own. Support emotionally and socially can be key. This is the role of family, friends, and support groups for those of us who are used to being in charge, this can be a difficult change. Now, we become reliant on family, friends, and caregivers, if for nothing else, but for support and understanding. Step by step, a little of the control of your life is given away. Adjustment is the process and adaption is how you get some control back.

Life without 'normal' vision is different. It is not so easy. Without complete vision you start noticing how inconvenient life can be. Things seem to take longer, require more effort, your responses are slower, and actions need to be more deliberate. You start concerning yourself about little stuff, with little fears about doing things, going places, and what others will think. Not to mention the new set of doctors and other eye care professionals. Now your 'business' becomes the business of educators, employers, and family and friends. Then there is the annoying and sometimes stupid stuff said by well meaning people, or people who just don't know any better. But it is not just the general public that doesn't get it; sometimes it is family and friends.

There will be those who don't really understand what is going on, and figure you have done well so far, and you will probably manage this well enough on your own. The truly clueless are those that are impatient or irritated by your incapability to do simple tasks (things you just can't see or don't understand because you can't see the details). They might be confused about what you can see and what you cannot see. Then there are those that are the complete opposite, that is, those who are trying to be very understanding and very helpful. They feel sorry for you, and feel they need to help 'poor you.' Somehow they must associate losing vision with losing brain cells, or they have some preconceived notions about blindness that are not applicable to you.

Whatever the relationship, others often do not understand how it is to function with vision loss. There needs to be a happy medium, where the family is understanding and helpful, to the extent that they have a vested interest in seeing you regain your sense of self-worth and independence, without making you feel helpless and dependent.

Although we may become consumed with our own grief and despair, we need to understand that our family members are also suffering a loss. Their lives change too. Whether it is a parent, child, or spouse, it can affect the family both emotionally and financially. The roles of the family members will change and financial burdens may increase and/or shift. The task of adjustment is not just for the visually impaired, but for all concerned.

Adjustment is the resetting of your life. This is what you have been handed, now what are you going to do? Adjustment, like acceptance, takes time. Adjustment is understanding that things must be done differently. Goals for schooling or employment will change. Activities you once enjoyed may change or be restricted. The independence you once commanded may now be curtailed. Adjustment is moving forward over all the hurdles of life. You may not be accepting of every change or challenge, but you just do the best you can do.

ADAPTION

Where there is a will there is a way.

There needs to be a willingness to believe that life will go on. It is that belief that gives you the hope to sustain a life of acceptance, adjustment, and adaption. It is what we do after we accept our disability that can make a difference. Acceptance, adjustment, and adaption are an ongoing process. Some will be able to work through this process to reclaim self-reliance. Some will never get to the point of acceptance.

Once you understand how your life will be different, now it is time to develop some skills of adaption. These are skills, techniques, some optical and others non-optical that will be compensatory. Once you have accepted the limitations, restrictions, and constraints, adaption is how you stay active mentally and engage in activities. Hopefully, independence, self-esteem, and satisfaction will follow as you find your new capability to function and maintain a good quality of life.

Among the issues to be addressed are: reading, activities of daily living, and independent mobility.

Some new skills you may slide into naturally. This is especially true for those who lose their vision in a slow progressive manner. Skills like eccentric fixation, head turns, scanning, and bringing things closer to enlarge images. But these adaptive skills may not come naturally to all visually impaired, especially those with sudden vision loss. These skills can be taught by an occupational or rehabilitation therapist who are trained to work with the visually impaired.

Activities of daily living modifications are made to make tasks easier that otherwise might take more time or impose limitations because of poor eyesight. Modifications are things like large print, better lighting, color coding, and organizing for easy accessibility. Changes are made not only to make life easier, but also for safety reasons. There are products that can be purchased in specialty stores, department stores, through catalog, or online. Things like big button phones or TV remotes, kitchen measuring utensils, talking thermometers, talking watches, and task lighting, along with a myriad of other gadgets, can be purchased to help around the home and office. Family members or a trained therapist can help with other home modifications for ease of use, organization, and safety.

When we think of vision loss, the first adaptive technique, most people recognize is magnification. The optical solutions take the form of strong eyeglasses, magnifying glasses, telescopes, and new and exciting electronic technologies. The choices are vast and appropriate selection can be confusing.

There are those aids that 'work' and those that do not 'work.' That variable depends on the individual and their type of vision loss. Often optical aids that are selected from department stores end up in the drawer. These magnifiers may be of poor quality, the wrong power, or are the wrong type for your needs. There are low vision specialists that can evaluate and recommend the right type and right power of optical aids. Low vision specialists can help with appropriate optical aids and technology.

If there is anything lucky about low vision at this time, it is that this is the age of computer technology. Computer software designers and cell phone manufacturers have realized the importance of accessibility and have created technology to help with nearly every aspect of life. "There's an app for that." Computer magnification programs, a CCTV, and e-books have made writing this book possible. It is this technology that can help those with disabilities to become educated and employed.

Here is the catch to adapting: You have to be willing to learn. It may take time and effort. It may not be easy and patience is required. You need to be your own advocate, because you may not be able to teach yourself skills and techniques of adaption. Don't be uncomfortable or embarrassed letting others know what you need. If they can't help you, there are professionals and agencies that can help you to solve problems.

Why You Should Seek a Low Vision Evaluation

The low vision evaluation is different from the medical eye examination that you receive from your optometrist or ophthalmologist. The medical examination is focused primarily on evaluating the health of the visual system, concluding with a diagnosis and subsequent treatment, if needed. The refraction, which determines the eyeglass prescription, is generally a part of that medical examination. Your eye doctor wants you to leave the office with the best vision possible.

If your vision is not optimal, in other words, not "20/20' with a new eyeglass prescription, additional testing will be done and a diagnosis determined. The doctor next considers the appropriate treatment, either medication or surgery. Sometimes there is no treatment, or the maximum treatment has been given, and there is no improvement in vision. The doctor may say 'nothing more can be done, see you in three months."

Nothing more can be done! This clinician may be brilliant within his/her scope of practice, but may not be aware of what the low vision specialist does, is too busy to concern himself, or may not be familiar with a referral network. They may think the patient is too old or the vision loss is too severe. I have heard of doctors, at the top of their profession, who send the patient out shopping for magnifiers.

This is where you need to be your own advocate. Low vision services can be found in private practices (optometrists or ophthalmologists who also practice low vision), low vision multidisciplinary centers, and state or federal agencies. Multidisciplinary low vision referral centers will have low vision specialists who work with occupational therapists, rehabilitation therapists, and counselors.

Low vision specialists are licensed optometrists or ophthalmologists, who understand the disease process and will have insight into the prognosis because of their medical training. They are knowledgeable about functional vision loss and understand their limitations. They have seen people with similar problems before, and will not think you are too old or too debilitated. Their goal is to help maximize your visual potential, and help you through the adjustment and adaption process.

The low vision specialist evaluates the type of vision loss, whether it is a loss of visual acuity, visual field, or contrast sensitivity, and then evaluates what visual function remains. Their goal is not to treat the disease process in a medical sense, as with medications or surgery. Medical treatment is still the domain of your regular eye doctor, with whom you should continue to see on a regular basis.

Here are the reasons to get a low vision evaluation;

1. To Advocate for Yourself;
2. Introduction to Visual Aids and Techniques;
3. Education and Counseling, and
4. Appropriate Referrals.

Advocating for Yourself

The low vision evaluation is your opportunity to interact with someone who understands your concerns and can answer your questions. The low vision specialist will delve into a detailed history looking for information about how you are functioning, your lifestyle, and personal needs. The evaluation needs to be interactive. Together, you and the doctor can set goals and create a plan to get you to where you need to be. This cannot be done effectively without a desire on your part to open up to new ideas. There needs to be acceptance on your part, a willingness to adjust your thinking, and an interest in adapting your life.

Introduction to Visual Aids and Visual Techniques

You have expressed concerns, interests, and lifestyle. The low vision specialist has gotten to know you. It is time to put away denial. If you are embarrassed or uncomfortable with using visual aids, put that away too. Visual aids help minimize the impact of your impairment.

The benefit of seeing a specialist is that he/she, because of knowledge and experience, can guide you in selecting the aids that would be helpful to you. They can match your needs for distance and near tasks with optical aids. Optical aids are those devices with lenses that help to enlarge or bring things closer. Unlike the department store, or online purchases, you can try them out. Beware of 'restocking fees' for return of products purchased online. The low vision specialist will guide you in their use.

Keep in mind, there is no one magical vision aid. Different tasks may each require a different device. (You may also notice that good quality visual aids are not cheap.) The low vision specialist or a rehabilitation specialist, will be able to instruct you in their use and other techniques of visual function.

Education and Initial Counseling

The initial low vision evaluation is usually a slow process, lasting anywhere from an hour to two hours. The low vision specialist will spend time explaining his/her findings along with an explanation of the recommendations. Prepare yourself for a very honest discussion about your impairment and options for rehabilitation. The discussion is tailored to you and your needs. This may also be the first person to give you some counseling regarding the social and psychological aspects of low vision.

There should be follow-up visits. The doctor is interested in your progress and can trouble-shoot any problems you may have. Low vision care will be ongoing, as your visual function and needs change.

Appropriate Referrals

The low vision specialist can also be the gateway to provide appropriate referrals to other professionals who work with the visually impaired. They often utilize the services of occupational therapists or rehabilitation specialists to teach visual skills, how to use visual aids, and skills of daily living. They typically are familiar with state and local agencies for educational services, social services, psychological counseling, and eligibility requirements. They may also know of support groups for those with similar vision losses.

Referrals: Rehabilitation Services

Rehabilitation services help to identify and train you in strategies and techniques useful to maximize remaining functional vision. Adaption is strengthened by training and use of compensatory skills. The goal is independence and some semblance of a normal life.

Therapists and specialists will introduce you to:

1. Reading and writing aids and techniques. Beyond the optical aids prescribed to you by the low vision specialist, they can help you select non-optical aids like large print materials, and advise you on audio reading options. There are also techniques for writing with assistive technologies both optical and non-optical.

2. Training in the use of optical aids, computer technology, and techniques such as eccentric fixation and scanning. You may benefit from instruction in use of the magnifiers prescribed by the low vision specialist. There are specific distances, ways of holding and moving the magnifier, which can make them easier to use. Some of the devices are electronic with different modes and options. A lesson from a therapist can help you learn to use these devices and computer technologies effectively. Eccentric fixation, scanning, and spotting are techniques they can teach you to use in order to maximize any residual vision.

3. Lighting, glare control, and contrast enhancement. The therapist will help with determining optimal lighting with lamps and light bulb options. They will also help with choices of illuminated non-optical aids. Those visually impaired who are sensitive to glare or who have problems with contrast will receive recommendations for filters.

4. Independent living. If needed, the therapist may make a visit to the home. Therapists assess the home for modifications for organization and safety. They can teach self reliant skills such

as cooking, management of housekeeping, self-grooming, and leisure activities. The goal is to make activities of daily living easier and safer.

5. Vocational (work) and educational (school). Therapists can recommend modifications to help with school and to keep you employed. Much of which involves technology to make assessable work and school related information. They may also know of additional state, federal, and private organizations that can help.

6. Orientation and Mobility. Orientation and mobility training is for independence and safety. The more severely impaired will require the help of an Orientation and Mobility Specialist. The goal is to help with independent movement around the house and in public. They can aid in helping the low vision patient in how to prevent falls and bumping into things. Training in orientation and mobility can also reduce the fear of getting lost, or finding ones way around in situations like shopping.

Referrals: Counseling Services

Psychiatric and social counseling is not found in every low vision center. This is the specialized area of psychiatrists, psychologists, and social workers. The loss of vision can be complicated by additional health concerns or there can be difficult family or living situations. Individuals working through these difficult issues may need the help of counselors above and beyond what the rehabilitation therapists are prepared to offer. If you need the help, your doctor, family, and friends may not identify this need. Remember to advocate for yourself. Vision loss can be a very painful and emotional mine field.

Why the Visually Impaired Refuse Optical and Non-Optical Aids

1. Denial. They truly believe they do not need any kind of visual aids. The reason why they don't see something is because it is too small, or it is somehow the fault of the thing they are trying to see. The other reason is the doctor, who they blame for not giving a very good prescription or something is wrong with the glasses. Using a visual aid is admitting they have a disability. There is no convincing them. They would rather give up activities (reading for example), than admit to needing help.

2. Depression. These are the people who have given up. They are not motivated to learn or to even try. They are not ready to accept the changes, and adjust their thinking. They are grieving their losses. Accepting the visual aid is another step to giving in to the disability. Psychosocial counseling is needed to help them move forward.

3. Resistance to New Things. This is a personality trait. Some people just assume it will be too difficult and they just don't feel they can devote any brain power to learning something that complicated or challenging. The hope is that they realize

that it is not really that tough, and it is well worth the time and effort.

4. Self-Image. The resistance to using visual aids is a part of their desire to appear 'normal'. They may find it embarrassing to draw attention to what is different about them, and fears that someone will start asking questions. Using a visual aid will stigmatize them as blind, a perception that can be damaging to the self esteem.

5. Previous Experience. While out shopping at the department store, or perhaps given to them by a well meaning family member, the visually impaired acquire magnifiers. They tried them, and they 'don't work.' Of course they don't work. Standing in a store, with bright fluorescent lights for two minutes, with what is probably an inexpensive magnifier designed for short-term spotting, is not the way to select a visual aid that can help you adapt. Department store magnifiers tend to be a lower power, and may not be the best optical grade.

6. Cost. During my career as an optometrist, I was always dazzled by patients that would buy a designer handbag but wouldn't spend the same amount of money on a pair of glasses that they put on their face every day. I was also puzzled by parents that took their kid to Disney World, but didn't want to spend a reasonable amount of money on good quality eyewear for the kid. Specialized visual aids are expensive, and you have to weigh cost vs. benefit. This is another reason for getting a low vision

evaluation. It gives you the opportunity to get professional guidance through the selection process and allows you to try them out in the office under more normal conditions. This may save you from making a costly mistake.

References:

1. Keeffe, Jill PhD. Vision Assessment and Prescription of Low Vision Devices. Community Eye Health. 2004; 17(49): 3–4.
2. Rosenthal, Bruce P. The Structured Low Vision Examination. Adapted from Problems in Optometry: A Structured Approach to Low Vision Care, Volume 3, Number 3, September 1991. Retrieved from **www.lighthouse.org**
3. Scheiman, Mitchell, Scheiman, Maxine, Whittaker, Stephen G. Low Vision Rehabilitation. A Practical Guide for Occupational Therapists. SLACK Incorporated, 2007.
4. Warren, Mary, OTP/L, SCLV,FAOTA, Baker-Nobles, Linda, MS, OY/L. Occupational Therapy Services for Persons with Visual Impairments. Retrieved from **www.ota.org**/ practioners/practiceareas./emergingareas/ PA/lowvision.aspx
5. VisionAware. vision Rehabilitation Services. Retrieved from **www.visionaware.org** › Everyday Living › Essential Skills.

CHAPTER 4

Adjusting to Vision Loss

Adjustment is the psychological and social resetting of your life. There are many factors that will affect how you adjust. Things like age of onset, rate and severity of disease progression, living situation, and financial concerns.

Coping is how we deal with the changes. It is how we adjust and adapt to the nuances of our psychological, social, and personal functional needs. An individual's coping mechanisms at the beginning of the disease are different from those at the various stages of the disease process. Someone who loses vision suddenly will need to overcome the shock of sudden disability, while someone with a slow, progressive onset of vision loss may have years to adjust and develop compensatory techniques. An individual with profound vision loss will need to work harder to compensate versus having to adapt to a milder vision impairment. One's living situation, whether living alone or in a family unit, can impact the capability to cope, depending on the situation, either positively or even negatively. Sadly, financial resources can impact the capability to cope. While state and federal agencies provide some valuable services, those extras like electronic technology, transportation, and home assistance may be financially out of reach.

There are several emotional issues that can affect one's capability to cope with a disability;

Grief

After the initial shock and realization that a most important aspect of your life is now disabled, grief floods in. The sense of loss is like losing a beloved family member. It can overwhelm you and leave you feeling like you are drowning in sadness, with no rescue in sight. Nothing will ever be the same.

It is said, that time heals all wounds. Perhaps, but vision loss is a wound we carry with us wherever we go, day in and day out. Give yourself permission to grieve. It is a normal part of adjusting to a disability. By denying it, grief can paralyze the coping process. The first step of acceptance is how we work through feelings of grief.

Depression

Depression is normal. It is more than just sadness. Depression can be mild, occasional episodes, or a severe daily occurrence. Persistent, functionally debilitating, long-term depression needs to be identified and addressed. The American Psychiatric Association (1) identifies major depression as having five of the following nine criteria:

1. Depressed mood such as feeling sad, empty, tearful, or irritable most of the day, nearly every day;

2. Decreased interest or pleasure in most activities, most of each day;
3. Significant weight change (5%) or change in appetite;
4. Change in sleep: Insomnia or increased interest in sleep;
5. Change in activity: restless or lethargic;
6. Fatigue or loss of energy;
7. Feelings of worthlessness or excessive or inappropriate guilt;
8. Find it difficult to think or concentrate or an inability to make decisions; and
9. Thoughts of death or suicide.

Loss of vision is a very emotional impairment. There is almost no aspect of life that it does not affect. Depression evolves from psychological and social changes. It hits at the perception of who you are and how you function. That in turn, affects how you interact with others and where you fit into the social structure.

Depression is not usually discussed in typical low vision services. But if not identified, adjustment and efforts to adapt will be unsuccessful. Advocate for yourself for mental health services if it is not offered to you. There is no shame in getting help. Depression is a well known aspect of acquired disability. Treatment can be an important step in regaining a sense of well-being and a good quality of life.

Negative Self-Perception

A negative self perception can affect your capability to cope. Perception of ourselves is often a reflection of how those around us perceive our disability. Family and friends may not understand, or are confused by what you are capable of seeing and doing. They may treat you differently than if you were fully sighted. Negative reactions by acquaintances and even strangers to low vision behaviors, things like getting close, wearing thick glasses or using a magnifier, can make you question yourself and impact your self-esteem and self confidence. Then there is the discomfort of having to explain to observers why you do what you do. A few embarrassing incidences may compel you to withdraw from social situations rather than enduring the humility of making what appears as a 'stupid' mistake.

Not seeing the details may mean that you miss out on the joke. Those with low vision may get left out of social activities which may require good vision or the need to drive. Feelings run to despair and loneliness, and strike at the perception of one's self-worth and self-confidence. Your impairment makes you feel conspicuous, and can result in social anxiety.

Stress

Mucking up the coping process is the burden of stress that a disability. brings with it. Like an unwelcome guest, it moves in with all its baggage and refuses to leave.

Stress associated with vision loss can come in many forms.

Stress starts with the knowledge that what you have is not curable. That can put anyone over the edge.

The feelings of how life could have, or should have been, are painful. Trying to keep life normal knowing that changes are out of your control is stressful.

All the negative feelings are their own source of stress. There can be overwhelming feelings of loss and fear. Depression, anxiety, and anger can wear you down and if too self-absorbed, these feeling can hinder your capability to cope. Everything is more difficult, takes longer, and puts a strain on you mentally.

The individual with a disability may not be able to earn as much money as before the disability, or may not be able to work at all. Consider how it can stress the family. It can change family dynamics. Roles within the family may perhaps shift. Loss of financial security and associated lifestyle changes puts stress on the family unit.

Loss of Independence

Loss or lack of independence can be a source of stress and depression. There is something to be said for being able to do what you want to do, when you want to do it, and how you want it done. Frustration and anger can arise with yourself or with others because you can't do or get something done because you just can't see well enough. Having to ask for help to read a menu, a sign, or needing help with self-grooming makes you feel helpless and out of control, which in turn degrades your feelings of self-sufficiency and self-worth.

The greatest symbol of independence is the capability to get into a car and drive off. Ask anyone who has not been able to get a driver's license or had to give theirs up. It is a tough blow to the psyche, especially as an American, not to have your 'wheels.' Having to rely on public transportation, if it is available, or always having to ask for transportation can be an added stress.

Limited capability to get around can leave the visually impaired isolated from spontaneous social interaction.

An Outline for Learning to Cope

Reduce Stress

Begin by identifying the problem areas. Not all problems will be solved, but accept that you will do what you can, within the framework of your situation.

The answer to reducing the financial stresses associated with a disability is outside my area of expertise. However, there are some things you can do to reduce the other associated stresses within your life. Here are a few suggestions:

Attitude Adjustment

Take a look at your attitude toward your impairment.

1. The Deniers. You can easily spot them because they are the excuse-makers. It is always the fault of something, or someone else in their mind. Deniers won't accept or deal with their loss and refuse to make the changes necessary to lead a new 'normal.'

These are the people who will not accept low vision devices. Often they live in the closet, meaning they don't tell others about their vision loss. The deniers may remain hopeful that a change in lifestyle will help or that a cure is just around the corner. They end up being frustrated, unhappy people. There are a lot of deniers out there. They need a reality check, and to seek the professional help needed to lead that normal life and to keep moving forward.

2. The Angry People. Life is a negative for them. They cannot get past the impairment to see that it is, what it is, and you can rant and rave, but it doesn't change anything. These people need to turn anger into action.

3. The Helpless. This individual feels so sorry for themselves, and languishes in their own helplessness. They are giving up, and look to others to make it make it easier for themselves. These individuals may realize the benefits of secondary gain. That is, their helplessness garners them more attention and concern from others. Family or friends that overindulge the helpless, are enabling them to remain helpless. The helpless can benefit from the professional help of rehab specialists and counselors.

4. The Resigners These are the people that sadly accept their impairment and shut down those more difficult parts of their life, assuming nothing can be done or it is just too hard. They live in mourning of their loss and unrelenting depression, "Woe is me," Eeyore. These people are part way there. They have accepted

their vision loss, now they need to do something about it to ensure a positive quality of life.

5. The Adapters. Finally, there are those that see their impairment as a challenge, and as something they just have to deal with. They have accepted it, they are adjusting, and are adapting. Life goes on. "Everybody's got somethin'." "What doesn't kill me makes me stronger." These individuals have a willingness to accept the help of low vision professionals and accessibility devices.

You might experience several different changes in attitude through the process of vision loss. Realize where you are emotionally, and set a goal to learn to accept, adjust, and adapt.

Social Interaction

The psychology of vision loss with its accompanied fears, social stigma, loss of independence, and depression can lead one to live a life in isolation. The less you interact with others the more inward you turn. Feelings of unhappiness, loss of self-worth, lack of self-esteem, lack of confidence, and that overwhelming sense of being alone, becomes magnified.

You are not alone. Even if you have a great family support system, communication with others with vision loss, or even other disabilities, is helpful in knowing how they are dealing with life. Family and friends may listen and try to understand your fears and concerns and try to help where they can. But be aware that there may be an expiration date on their capability to listen to complaints, rants, whining, and demands on their time. They love you, but...

Talking with others can help you sort out your own feelings. Support groups were created for this reason. Commiserating with others, listening to how they cope, learning that their fears are similar to yours, and that you are not so unusual.

If support groups are not your thing, consider talking to others who have disabilities other than vision impairment. Often those with vision impairments don't know anyone else with vision problems. There is a common thread among those with disabilities regarding psychological and social issues. Even if you think you have nothing in common with others, friendships can be built by sharing war stories of disability challenges. You can learn from others with disabilities, not only about how to cope, but about your own strengths and weaknesses.

If your living situation is one in which you cannot access outside support, online message boards and blogs related to various types of low vision and even specific eye diseases are out there. It can be helpful just to be able to read about someone else with the same concerns as you. These sites are also a good source of coping information.

Engage Your Mind

Do you wake up in the morning and drag around the house, really not getting anything done. So you turn on the TV, thinking "I'm doing something....I'm watching or listening to TV." Ok, that good for awhile, then what?

Self-help advocates will tell you that to feel self-worth and satisfaction we need to feel a purpose. Setting goals, creating things (work), hobbies, activities both physical and mental, and responsibilities, can help fend off feelings of despair. You will not completely forget your disability, as a matter of fact, it will emerge to remind you of its presence throughout the day, but it is how you deal with it that is a measure of your capability to cope.

Knowledge is Power

I have always believed in knowledge as a source of power. The more you learn and the more you know, that information can make a big difference. A college professor once said to me that you can argue any point with your professor, if you do your homework. I am not saying that you need to become an expert in the field of low vision or the medical nuances of your particular disease, but you can learn to understand the disability, its impact on your visual function, and how to compensate. You can best help yourself by learning how to help yourself.

The information is out there, more so than it has ever been in history. Assistive technology is far more sophisticated and accessible than ever. Public understanding, although it still has a ways to go, is opening up opportunities for those with disabilities.

"Ask, and it will be given to you; seek, and you will find; knock, and it will be opened to you." Matthew 7:7 New King James Bible.

Seek the Help of Professionals

No one out there knows or understands it all. There is a specialty for nearly every associated issue of disability. These professionals each have an area of expertise to offer. Your needs will change as you reorganize your life and deal with the psychological and social issuers.

A good source of information is the low vision specialist team. They are often knowledgeable about state agencies, community support groups, and organizations that offer help to those with disabilities. You just need to know about them in order to find them and access their services. The person best qualified to advocate for you is you!

Humor

Years ago, I listened to a pop-culture self-help CD in which a woman said she helped herself through cancer by watching funny movies and making sure she laughed all day. Well, I don't know about laughter curing cancer, but I do believe it is good for the soul.

While it is easy to allow all the negative emotions that come along with a life disabled, lifting ourselves up is much harder. Maintaining a sense of humor does not mean that you need to come up with a comedy routine, but it is a mind set of having the capability to put the negative thoughts aside and opening yourself up to the humor of life's situations. It can mean looking for enjoyment and pleasure in life, whether it is a stress releasing activity, a positive friendship, loving pets, or enjoyable entertainment. Seek out those things that make you smile and laugh.

You need to remember that you are not a disability, but the impairment is only a part of who you are. You are still a normal person, who can enjoy life, and have a good laugh. Try to start by not taking yourself too seriously and opening yourself up to positive thoughts. Be able to laugh at yourself, even if it is not out loud.

Conclusion

In a phrase, focus on ability not disability.

The process of learning to cope is a long one. Adjusting to the psychological and social changes is a stepwise process. While many factors may seem to be insurmountable, you need to identify and address these issues. Advocate for yourself by stating the problem, seeking help, and asking the questions. There is no assurance that all problems will be solved, but as my father use to say "You don't know, unless you ask."

Additional Reading

Reinhardt, Joann P. PhD; Horowitz, Amy DSW/PhD; and Sussman-Skalka, Carol **J.LMSW**, MBA. Depression, Vision Loss and Vision Rehabilitation. Lighthouse International, **www.lighthouse.org** Home > Services & Assistance > Social Services > **Depression, Vision Loss and Vision Rehabilitation**.

References

1. Diagnostic and Statistical Manual of Mental Disorders (DSM) 5th Ed., published by the American Psychiatric Association. Diagnostic Criteria for Major Depressive Disorder and Depressive Episodes American Psychiatric Publishing, Incorporated 2013.
2. Fox, Steven. Visual Impairment: Understanding the Psychosocial Impact. An Expert Interview With Khadija S. Shahid, OD, FAAO. Medscape Multispecialty. October 29, 2012.
3. Moran, Carmen C., Beyond Content: Does Using Humor help Coping? Disabilities Studies Quarterly. Volume 23, No. 3/4, Summer/ Fall 2003. <www.dsq-sds.org>
4. Scheiman, Nitchell, OD,FCOVD,FAAO, Scheiman Maxine MEd, OTR/L,CLVTWhittaker, Stephen G. PhD, OTR/L, CLVT. Psychosocial Issues Related to Visual Impairment, Low Vision Rehabilitation A Practical Guide for Occupational Therapists, SLACK Incorporated, Memphis, TN pg 83-88.
5. Wolffe, Karen E., Adults with Low Vision: Personal, Social and Independent Living Needs. Foundations of Low Vision: Clinical and Functional Perspectives. AFB Press, New York, pg.322=339.
6. Zell Sacks, Sharon. Psychological and social Implications of Low Vision. Foundations of Low Vision: Clinical and Functional Perspectives. AFB Press, New York, pg. 26-41.

CHAPTER 5

The Low Vision Team

There is frequent confusion in the public mind as to who performs eye examinations, treats eye disease, and who makes eyeglasses. Although there is overlap in some of these job descriptions, each professional plays a part in eye care or rehabilitative services in which they excel.

Optometrist (OD)

The practice of optometry has evolved over the last 20 years, from being just refractionists (those who determine eyeglass prescriptions) to primary eye care providers. State laws have changed, allowing optometrists to expand their scope of practice. They perform routine eye examinations not just to calculate an eyeglass prescription, but also to diagnose eye disease and provide treatment. Optometrists are experts in contact lens fitting and care. The practice of optometry has always included a special interest in low vision and binocular vision. Because of their training in optics, optometrists have long been the source for visual aids by those with subnormal vision and vision therapy for disorders of binocular function.

Education

Optometrists have a bachelor's degree from an accredited college, typically with an emphasis on basic science, biology, chemistry, mathematics, and physics. Four more years are spent in optometry school. Courses include optics, visual perception, anatomy, pathology, pharmacology, psychology, neuro-anatomy, neuro-physiology, and binocular vision. More specialized courses include contact lens fitting, opticianry, and low vision. One year is spent as an extern in a primary care facility like a clinic, hospital, or a referral center, seeing and treating patients. Some optometrists chose to go on to a residency program.

When their education is complete, each optometrist must take a comprehensive national board examination, plus a state licensing written and practical examination.

Low Vision Specialist

A low vision specialist is either an optometrist or ophthalmologist. Optometrists focus much of their training on the mathematics and physics of optical lenses and the eye. This specialized training makes them well qualified to prescribe visual aids that help those with sub-normal vision.

Low vision specialists usually work on a referral basis, from other eye care providers. They also make recommendations for referrals to other members of the low vision rehabilitation team based on their assessment of the low vision patient's needs

Ophthalmologists (MD)

Ophthalmologists are medical doctors who, after completing medical school and a one year internship, go on to do three years of a hospital-based ophthalmology residency. Even beyond those three years they can specialize as corneal specialists, vitreo-retinal specialists, neuro-ophthalmologists, oculo-plastic surgeons, glaucoma specialists, and pediatric ophthalmologists.

The overlap between optometrists and ophthalmologists is that they both do primary eye care, however, ophthalmologists are specialized as surgeons. Because they are surgeons and can provide advanced treatment, many patients are referred to them for secondary care.

Opticians (LO)

Opticians are responsible for filling eyeglass and contact lens prescriptions written by the optometrists or ophthalmologists. They are the ones behind the glass windows edging lenses and assembling eyeglasses. Opticians are pros at knowing materials and products of the eye care business. They help with frame selection, making lens choice recommendations, measuring, fitting, and dispensing eye wear.

They attend a one or two year program, do an internship in an opticianry, and some states require a licensing examination.

Where they overlap with optometrists is contact lens fitting, and some states allow them to refract.

Dispensing opticians can work as independents with their own optical shop, or in the opticianry as an employee of an optometrist or ophthalmologist, or for one of the large retail chains.

Therapists and Specialists for Low Vision

Low vision care can extend beyond the low vision clinician (optometrist or ophthalmologist), to include a team of rehabilitation therapists, trained to work with the visually impaired based on the findings of the low vision evaluation.

Rehabilitation refers to the education and training of the visually impaired in the use of visual aids and implementation of strategies and techniques to maximize the potential to function as independently as possible, despite the impairment.

There are several different certified therapist and specialists, with some overlap in their roles. But each serves a vital role in the rehabilitation plan, with some differences in specialty. Which of these therapists you see, will be determined by the doctor, clinician, facility, or agency making the referral.

Low Vision Therapist (CLVT)

The Certified Low Vision Therapist works in conjunction with the optometrist or ophthalmologist low vision specialist. They help with training you in the use of the low vision aids prescribed by the doctor. They educate patients as to the optical and non-optical adaptive aids and make additional recommendations. They can teach the visual skills needed to maximize the use of remaining vision and other compensatory skills , such as non-visual techniques, with an emphasis on using other senses. Low vision therapists educate family and caretakers and help them understand the patient's visual function and expectations during the rehabilitative process.(1)

To learn more about the scope of practice of a Low Vision Therapist, check the ACVREP website: **www.acvrep.org.** Certified Low Vision Therapist (CLVT) Handbook Section2 Scope of Practice

Vision Rehabilitation Therapist (CVRT)

Certified Vision Rehabilitation Therapists provide a more in-depth instruction in activities of daily living, computer accessibility, home life management, and leisure activities. They assess the home, work, and educational needs, and instruct the visually impaired that may have other disabilities, as to coping strategies in these areas of their life. Rehabilitation therapists also evaluate the psychosocial implications of the individual's disability. These therapists can make referrals to other therapists, specialists, and counselors, based on their assessment.(2)

To learn more about the certification if a Rehabilitation Therapist, visit the website: **www.acvrep.org** Certified Vision Rehabilitation Therapist (CVRT).

Occupational Therapist (OT)

Occupational therapists are "experts in activity analysis and environmental modification."(3) They evaluate the work, home, and educational environment and assess the limitations imposed by the individual's impairment, and develop strategies for the visually impaired to cope. They are also trained to assess and make recommendations for limitations imposed by other disabilities. The occupational therapist then trains the impaired in adaptive techniques using optical and non-optical aids which specifically address their needs. This evaluation and assessment may involve a trip on the part of the OT, to the home or workplace of the low vision patient.

To learn more about Occupational Therapists, visit the Association of Occupational Therapy Association website: **www.aota.org** About-Occupational-Therapy.

Orientation and Mobility Specialists (COMS)

Certified Orientation and Mobility Specialists help the visually impaired with strategies for movement indoors and outdoors. This is a service usually required for the more severely impaired. These specialists train the visually impaired to use their senses and any remaining vision, and in the use of a cane. The orientation and mobility specialist evaluates the home and workplace for safety and ease of movement and uses this information to help the individual use cues and senses to orient themselves and successfully move around. Orientation and mobility training can help the impaired with navigating through urban areas, such as streets and public transportation. The skills taught by an orientation and mobility specialist will help with the confidence, independence, and safety of the visually impaired.(4)

To learn more about the scope of practice of an Orientation and Mobility Specialist, visit **www.acvrep.org.** Certified Orientation and Mobility Specialist (COMS) Handbook Section 2

Teachers of the Visually Impaired

Teachers of the visually impaired use the diagnosis along with other information provided to them from other specialists and therapists and do their own functional assessment in the school environment. They become the student's advocate. by interpreting the medical information and understanding the needs of the individual low vision student. They relay this information to the educational team to assure the student has access to academic learning.(5)

Rehabilitation Counselors

Rehabilitation counselors will guide and coordinate rehabilitation services. They often determine eligibility for services by virtue of the disability and economic need. They will oversee job skill development and a subsequent job search. Essentially they are case managers who counsel and advocate between agencies for the disabled.(6)

Accessing Services

Eye Examinations:

- **American Optometric Association** via the **Bright Focus** website: Select zip code to search. **www.brightfocus.org/**
- **American Academy of Ophthalmologists**, The Eye MD Association **https://secure.aao.org/aao/find-an-eye-md**.
- **WebMD** website**,** Find a Doctor, Physicians Directory **doctor.webmd.com/You** can find eye care groups and MD's by specialty
- **Find A Doctor** website **https://www.findadoctor.com/** Optometrists and Ophthalmologists can be found by city or zip code.

Finding Low Vision Services

Each state has a Department of Rehabilitation and/or a Commission for the Blind and Visually Impaired. Here is how to find those resources in your state:

- **American Federation for the Blind**
  website: **http://www.afb.org**
  Home > Programs & Services > Our Family of Websites

  Scroll to Directory of Services (on the right side) with the 'Find Local Services' dropdown menu. (Not the Directory Center) If you type in your state, a list of types of services comes up. Low Vision is one of them. Select the service and a list of all your state's organizations that provide the services you are looking for pops up. This list includes not only state government resources, but local organizations. Addresses and phone numbers are included. If you click on the organization, a description of their services comes up. This is a **very** good resource.

OR

- **VisionAware**
  http://www.visionaware.org
  or **visionaware@afb.net**

  This is one of the AFB websites. Scroll down to "Looking for help" (lower right side). Fill in your state name, and a list of state and private organizations comes up. This is another really good website. VisionConnect is their accessible directory of services app.

- **National Council of State Agencies for the Blind**
  NCSAB Directory http://www.ncsab.org
  This is a very easy access to the contact information of your state's department for low vision services / rehabilitation serves. Just click on your state's two letter abbreviation and the listing comes up.

Rehabilitative Services:

- **American Optometric Association** via the **Bright Focus** website, **www.brightfocus.org**.

Find an Optometrist. Select for Rehabilitation services (at the bottom), for a selected zip code.

- **Lions Club**
  Lions Clubs are community-based, volunteer service organizations. The Lions are Helen Keller's "Knights of the blind in the crusade against darkness." The Lions Clubs have numerous programs in support of vision, hearing, heath, and youth services. Individual clubs may vary in their focus. There are Lions Club Low Vision Centers and low vision centers supported by the Lions, which offer education and rehabilitative services. Check with your local Lions Club or check the previously mentioned AFB Directory of Services webpage for your state.

Financial Help

- **Benefits.gov** Your Path to Government Benefits govbenefits.gov/
  This website has a questionnaire format calculator to guide you in determining if you are eligible for government benefits. There is an easy to follow questionnaire.
- **Social Security Administration http://www.ssa.gov/disability/**
  This website has a Benefits Eligibity Tool if you are thinking about applying for Social Security benefits. This site has information on applying for benefits and the forms needed. There are also phone numbers to call to apply.

- **EyeCare America** On line referral webpage: **www.eyecareamerica.org/**
  EyeCare America is the public service program of the Foundation of the American Academy of Ophthalmologists. This is the Online referral site for free eye exams by volunteers. There is an online questionnaire to determine eligibility.
- **Optometry Cares; The AOA Foundation** www.optometryscharity.org/vision-usa/ Vision USA Optometry Cares Foundation. Through the foundation those who qualify as low-income can get free eye exams. In order to access Vision USA services, an online application must be submitted on your behalf by a social worker, charitable organization,or agency.
- **New Eyes for the Needy**
  www.new-eyes.org/>>Apply for a Voucher
  This is a national organization that is able to help low-income individuals get free eyeglasses. The applicant must have a recent eyeglass prescription. A voucher must be applied for on your behalf by a social services agency or a school nurse. The voucher can then be taken to a participating eyeglass dispensary. The organization does not help with eye examinations.
- **One Sight** https://onesight.org/
  Taken from their website: " To be eligible for our voucher services, please partner with a 501(c)3 non-profit

organization like the American Red Cross, Lion's Club, Prevent Blindness or other social agency in your community. Once verified, they can provide you with a referral letter that can be taken to a local LensCrafters, Pearle Vision, Sears Optical, or Target Optical location. Store associates can assist you in obtaining eyewear."

References

1. Certified Low Vision Therapist (CLVT) Handbook, Section 2 - Scope of Practice for Low Vision Therapists. Retrieved from: **www.acvrep.org**.
2. Certified Vision Rehabilitation Therapist (CVRT) **www.acvrep.org**.
3. Warren, Mary, OTR/R, SLLV, EAOTA, Baker Nobles, Linda. MS, OT/L. Occupational Therapy Services for Persons with Visual Impairments.
4. Certified Orientation and Mobility Specialist (COMS) Handbook, Section 2 - Scope of Practice for Orientation and Mobility Certification. Retrieved from: **www.acvrep.org**.
5. Corn, Anne L., Koenig, Alan J., Foundations of Low Vision: Clinical and Functional perspectives, AFB press, 2000, Pg. 186.
6. Scope of Practice. American Rehabilitation Counseling Association. Retrieved from: **www.arcaweb.org/**.

CHAPTER 6

The Eye Examination

An eye examination should be a standard part of routine medical care. The American Optometric Association recommends routine eye exams every 2 years for adult ages 18 to 60 years old, and every year after 61. (1) Routine eye care is essential for those with risk factors such as medical conditions, like diabetes, a family history of eye disease such as glaucoma, and those with exposure to environment factors known to cause eye disease such as smoking and high UV light exposure.

Good eyesight is not the sole indicator of eye health. Early onset of potentially blinding eye disease can be picked up during the routine eye examination. The doctor gathers baseline information and a determination of diagnosis is made. Treatment may be as simple as a set of eyeglasses or more critically sight saving, involving medications or surgery. Eye examination data passed on to low vision and rehabilitation specialists will help to guide the course of low vision rehabilitation.

Step 1: The History

Even before the doctor asks any questions, he or she has already begun the exam by observation. The doctor is observing the eyes as to their appearance. Do they look the same? Are they red or irritated? Are they aligned? How do they move? Also, does the patient tilt or turn their head when observing the doctor? Does the patient have any repetitive movements, like rubbing, blinking, or any ticks?

The doctor wants to know about the history of your current problem. Things like;

- When did it start?
- How long does it last?
- How frequent?
- Any other associated signs, symptoms or changes?
- Has anything relieved the problem?
- Any compensatory actions you have taken?
- Have you experienced this before?

This last question now leads into your eye history. If the technician hasn't already addressed it, the examiner needs to know about eye wear, glasses, and contact lenses. It is important to tell the doctor of any eye surgeries you might have had, including those as a child. The doctor would also like to know of eye medications you have taken, trauma you have experienced, or any vision therapy done in the past. Significant eye history of blood relatives, especially mother, father, brothers, and sisters, is relevant. Family eye history can indicate a risk for some eye diseases.

The eye can mirror systemic disease. The doctor is interested in your general medical history. Diseases of the cardiovascular system, neurological diseases, autoimmune diseases, hereditary disorders, and trauma can all have an impact on the future of your vision. What medication we take is an important part of our medical history. Medications can affect our vision, possibility causing mild side effects like dryness or blurring, to more serious conditions like cataracts.

The doctor, by virtue of the initial observation and history, has already begun to form a mental checklist of a possible diagnosis. Now the rest of the exam is the testing that will help the doctor confirm or rule out a possible diagnosis. The importance of history cannot be underestimated.

Step 2: Tests of Visual Function

Visual Acuity

Visual acuity is a measurement of central vision capability. Attaching numbers to the measurement is a way to quantify the capability to see fine line and detail. There are numerous ways to test visual acuity. The most commonly used is the Snellen chart. This is the one that uses the 20 foot notation, and is associated with the big E as the 20/400 letter at the top of the chart. This test uses the highest contrast, that is, black on white. Because it is high contrast, problems with glare and low contrast sensitivity will not be identified. It is the job of the low vision specialist to evaluate these other problems.

The notation 20/20 means that at 20 feet (test distance is indicated by the first number) a normally sighted person should be able to see a letter 8.7mm in height. The second half of the measurement is based on this as a starting point. For example, the 'legal' blindness designation of 20/200 means that at 20 feet. a letter must be 10 times larger (200 divided by 20 = 10), or 87 mm (8.7 mm x 10 = 87 mm or 8.7 cm) in order to be identified by a person with the 20/200 vision impairment. Another way to describe the notation is that the person with 20/200 vision needs to see at the closer distance of 20 feet what the 'normal' sighted person can see at 200 feet.

Another example is a person with 20/50 needs a letter that is 21.75 mm (or 2.175 cm) at 20 feet to be able to identify it. Calculated as: 50 divided by 20 = 2.5 , then calculate: 2.5 x 8.7 mm = 21.75 mm. Or the person with 20/50 vision needs the closer distance of 20 feet, to see what the 'normal' person can see at 50 feet.

Occasionally, if a patient is unable to read the 20/40 line, even with their best set of eyeglasses, the doctor will place a paddle with pinholes in front of the eye. The patient is asked to peer through one of the pinholes to see. What the pinhole does is focus the light rays on the back of the eye. The visual acuity is retested and If the patient sees better, this indicates that a prescription change is in order. If there is no improvement in what is seen, this indicates to the doctor that there is most likely some vision problem that cannot be corrected with a change in eyeglass prescription. Appropriately enough this is called the pinhole test.

The measurement of visual acuity is a very important key to how the rest of the examination will progress.

The Rapid Neurological Tests:

1. Pupil Measurement

   A penlight is shone alternately between the two eyes. The doctor is looking at the size, shape, and reactivity of the pupils. Differences in size or reactivity can indicate a problem in the innervations to the pupil, or optic nerve damage secondary to trauma or disease.

2. Eye Muscle Movement

   This test is done by having the patient follow (with eye movement only) a small object, either in a letter H shape or a circle. The doctor is watching to see if both eyes move smoothly, accurately, fully, and equally. It is important to note any pulling or double vision as the eyes move outward. This is a neurological test of muscle function.

3. Visual Field Screening

   This is just a quick check for a defect of the nerves responsible for peripheral vision. The doctor sits across from the patient, and asks the patient to fixate on the doctor's eye. In the side vision, the doctor will hold up fingers (finger-counting visual fields), a small object, or a penlight. The patient is asked to identify where in their side vision the object, fingers, or light is located, without looking in that direction. It is not a very sensitive test, but can alert the doctor to a significant visual field loss and indicate the need for further testing.

There are a few other screening tests that the doctor may opt to perform:

4. Color Vision Screening

   It is good to document any color vision deficiencies. Some eye diseases can change color vision perception, so it is important to have baseline data as to whether or not a patient has a hereditary or acquired (through disease) form of color deficiency.

   The most common color vision test used is the Ishihara test. The individual Ishihara test plates are a circle filled with small individually colored circles. A person with normal color vision will see a pattern. The capability to see the pattern, and identify that pattern as a number, means the patient is able to discriminate colors. The Ishihara test identifies the color deficiencies of the red-green type, which is the most common type of inherited color deficiency.

5. Amsler Grid

   This is a test for the function of the central 10 degrees of vision. If a doctor does not see an improvement in vision with the pinhole test, he or she may opt to do an Amsler grid. This test may be performed routinely on older patients. Often a copy of the grid is given to them to take home as a means to monitor their own vision.

   Amsler grid will be discussed more thoroughly in the low vision examination section.

6. Stereopsis (Depth Perception)

   This test for depth perception is occasionally done on adults, but is more commonly done with children. Stereopsis testing measures the patient's capability to detect small degrees of separation, and tells the doctor if the two eyes are working together. Testing is done with a special booklet (Stereo Fly or Wirt 4 dot) in combination with tinted polarized lenses. (Similar to the 'glasses' used to view 3D movies.) The polarization of the eye lenses are aligned at different angles to give the two eyes a slightly different image. A person with good depth perception will see that the objects in the booklet appear to stand off the page, as if 3 dimensional. Depth perception is measured by degree of separation of the two images, as detected by the patient.

Step 3: Refraction

Refraction is the determination of the corrective eyeglass lenses required by the patient to see most clearly. The doctor uses a phoroptor. The phoroptor is the instrument that is moved into position in front of the patient's face, with the viewing apertures in front of both eyes. It has many lenses which can be presented to the patient in innumerable combinations. The doctor begins with a starting point, determined by objective findings. Objective findings are a starting point determined without the patient's input. Doctors will use an auto-refractor or a retinoscope light to take initial measurements. Then the testing becomes interactive. The doctor will refine the prescription by using a series of choices. (One better or two?) The final, best correction is achieved in a step-wise manner.

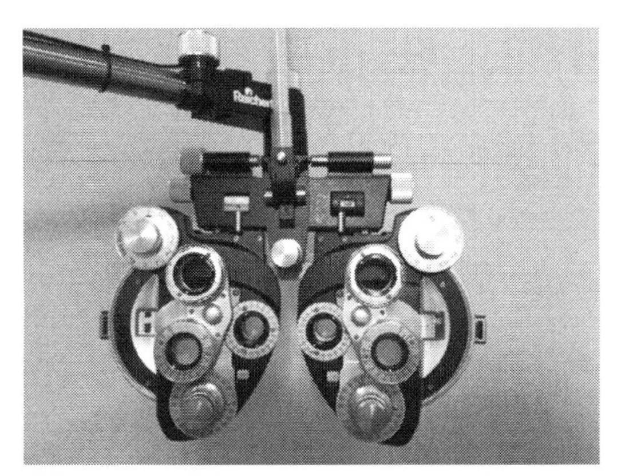

Photo: Phoropter, used to determine the eyeglass prescription.

Step 4: The Health Assessment

The final phase of the routine examination is an evaluation of the health of the eyes.

1. Slit Lamp Examination

   The slit lamp is the instrument set on the moveable table. It is placed in front of the patient. The head must be placed on the chin rest and the forehead should be resting against the upper band. The slit lamp is a microscope to magnify the front of the eye. The doctor is able to evaluate the details of the lids, lashes, conjunctiva, cornea, and iris (collectively known as the anterior segment of the eye). Using additional lenses, the slit lamp can also be used to peer into the back of the dilated eye (referred to as the posterior segment). The slit lamp can be modified with lasers for treatment or by adding a camera for photographing the eye.

2. Tonometry

The slit lamp may also have an attached tonometer to measure eye pressure. It is the cone-shaped lens on a stem that glows a cobalt blue. In order to visualize the cornea, and take the measurement, a drop of fluorescein dye is placed in the eye. This technique of eye pressure measurement has become more favored by professionals over the older 'puff of air' test.

The reason for eye pressure measurement is to determine the patients risk for developing the eye disease called glaucoma. An acceptable eye pressure measurement can vary from person to person. A general guideline is 8 to 21 mmHg. Rarely is one pressure measurement diagnostic of glaucoma. It may be a series of measurements, or additional testing that finalizes a diagnosis of glaucoma.

Photos:

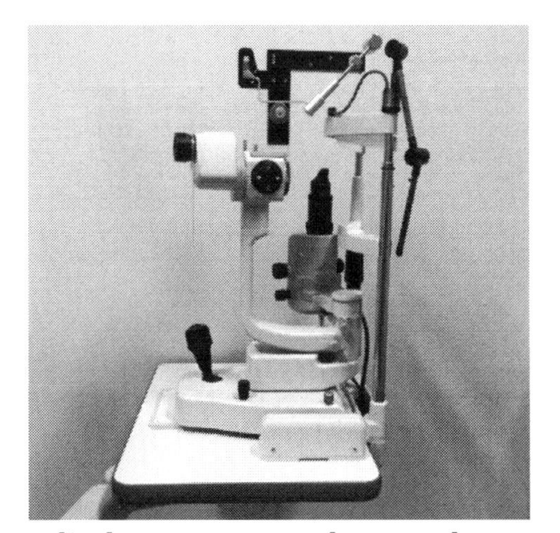

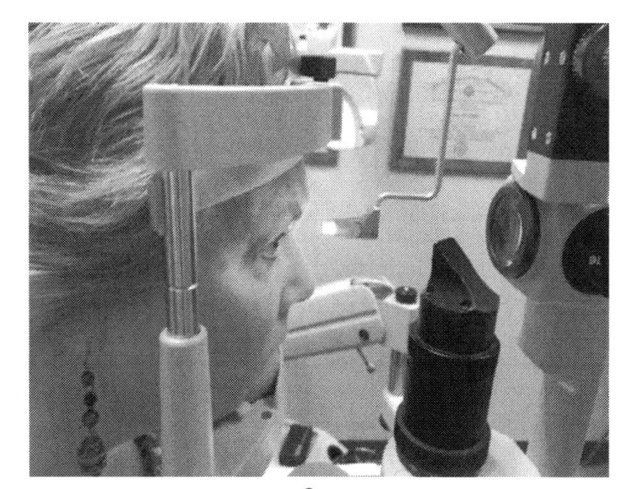

Slit lamp to evaluate the eye, tonometry test for eye pressure.

3. Dilated Fundus Examination

   A comprehensive eye examination includes dilation of the pupil for evaluation of the posterior segment of the eye. Drops called mydriatics act to relax both the iris muscle and the muscle responsible for the ability to focus. That is why the patient becomes both light sensitive and experiences blurred vision. Because bright lights are needed to peer into the dark chiasm of the eye, and the eyes' natural reaction is for the pupil to clamp down to as small an opening as possible, dilation is necessary. A thorough evaluation cannot be done through a normally small pupil opening. The dilation solves the problem, and without focusing capability, it makes it somewhat more tolerable for the patient.

   The slit lamp can be used once again in combination with additional lenses to view the back of the eye. An evaluation of the lens of the eye for cataracts is done at this point.

   The doctor may also select a small hand held instrument called an ophthalmoscope. The doctor comes in very close to get a detailed look at the posterior retina, macula, and optic nerve. The other instrument used is an indirect ophthalmoscope. This instrument has ocular lenses and is mounted on the doctor's head. The doctor next uses hand held lenses, and in effect makes like a telescope to view the far peripheral areas of the retina not seen with the other instruments.

Other Common Testing Procedures

1. Automated Visual Field

   The inside of this instrument is shaped like a bowl to mirror the bowl shaped interior of the eye. The visual acuity test and the refraction have determined the function of the central visual area. The purpose of the visual field test is to determine the function of the rest of the retina. A patient can have 20/20 vision centrally, and still have significant visual field loss.

   Once again the patient's chin is placed on the chin rest, and the forehead is resting against the upper band. One eye is patched, and the patient is given a 'clicker' with a button on it to communicate their answers with the computer. The instruction is to keep the central vision focused on a small lit diode. The automated program presents small flashes of light, often at different light intensities, in a grid pattern on the inside of the bowl. When the light flash is seen in the patient's peripheral field of vision, they respond with a touch of the button. The instrument is pretty smart. It will notify the tester if the patient starts looking around, or shifts positron. The person administering the test can also observe what the patient is doing by looking at the closed circuit camera display! What the doctor is looking for are areas of either loss vision (absolute scotomas) or areas that are just less sensitive (relative scotomas).

Photos:

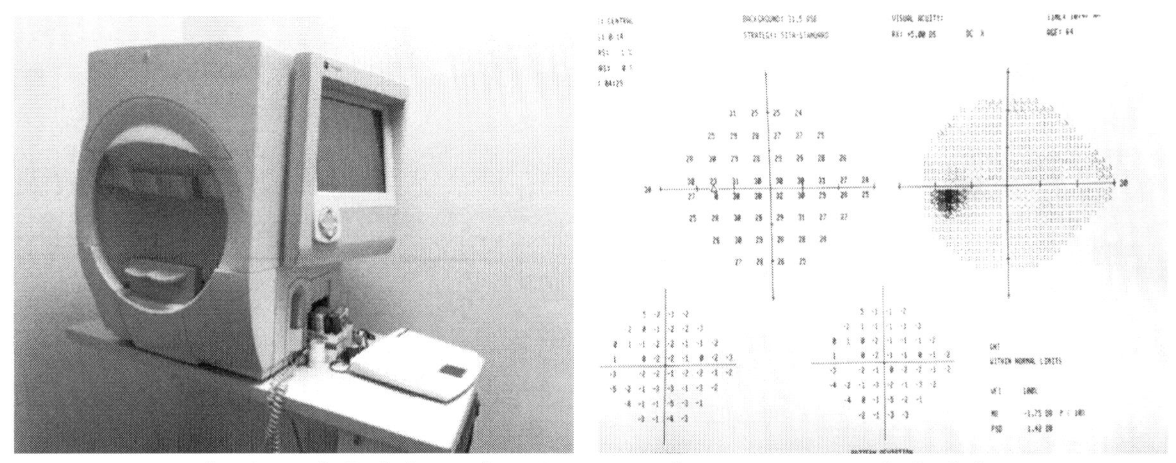

Automated visual field and Print out from a visual field test

2. Ocular Coherence Tomography (OCT)

This is truly an amazing piece of technology. An OCT scan is a method of imaging the retina, in the back of the eye, to give the doctor a 2 dimensional cross sectional view that reveals microscopic details that cannot be seen by the human eye. This technology can detect eye disease at a much earlier stage than before.

Best part of all for the patient is that there is no special preparation. The test is analogous to a non-invasive, non-contact biopsy of the human retina. This technology uses light that is non-damaging to the retina. The light seen by the patient is in the near infrared wavelength. The OCT analyses how the individual layers of the retina reflect these light scans back to the instrument. Some retinal layers are more reflective than others, and some reflect very little. Damage or defects can be seen as breaks in the pattern of these layers of the retina. (2)

The patient places their chin in the chin rest, with their forehead against the upper band. A steady head position and an eye with steady fixation are essential. The quality of the image is dependent on the patient remaining still. The operator aligns the eye, and then will ask the patient not to blink. A good 2 seconds of good fixation and no movement is required. What the patient sees is patterns of red lines in a star or circle formation. That's it! The computer calculates retinal thickness, and produces a cross-sectional image of the retina. Additionally, with this information, it can build a 3 dimensional image. What can now be viewed is what is going on within the retina or just below the surface; things like tissue loss, fluid, and detachments are now visible.

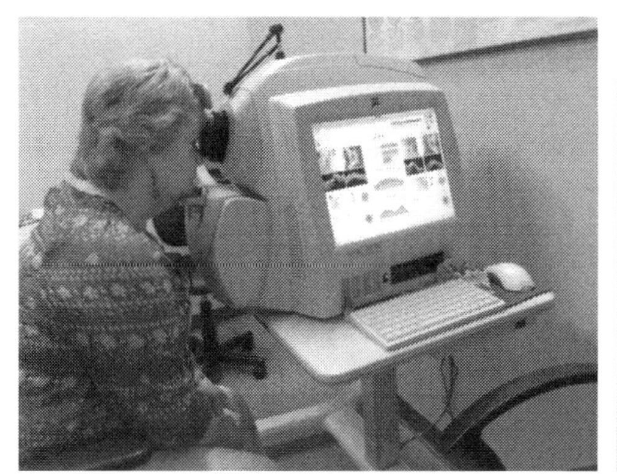

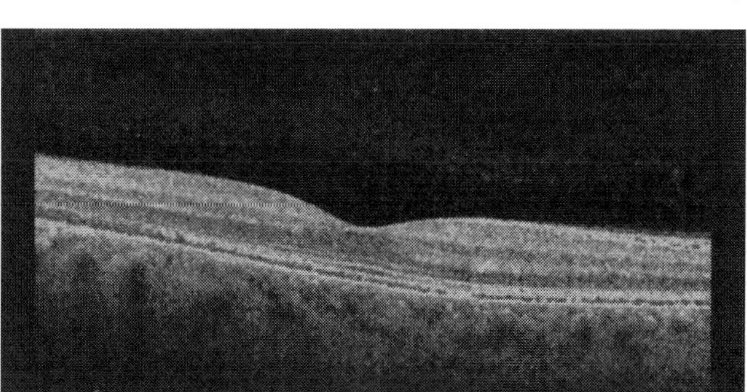

Photos: OCT instrument and a Scan showing layers of the retina

3. Fluorescein Angiography

While the OCT is looking at the thickness and integrity of the retinal tissue, the fluorescein angiography is performed to look at the blood circulation to the retina and the choroid below. Besides being dilated, the patient will receive an injection of fluorescein dye. The camera uses black and white slides to take a series of photographs to document the passage of the dye through the retinal and choroidal vasculature.

The patient places their chin in the chin rest and the forehead against the upper band to keep the head steady and in position. A qualified person will inject the arm with the fluorescein dye. Knowing how long it takes the dye to get from the arm to the eye, 9 to 10 seconds, the photo series begins, at a rate of 1 photo (accompanied with a flash) per second, for 20 seconds. There is a very predictable pattern of blood flow. What the doctor is looking for is leakage, blockage, pooling of blood, and any abnormal blood vessels.

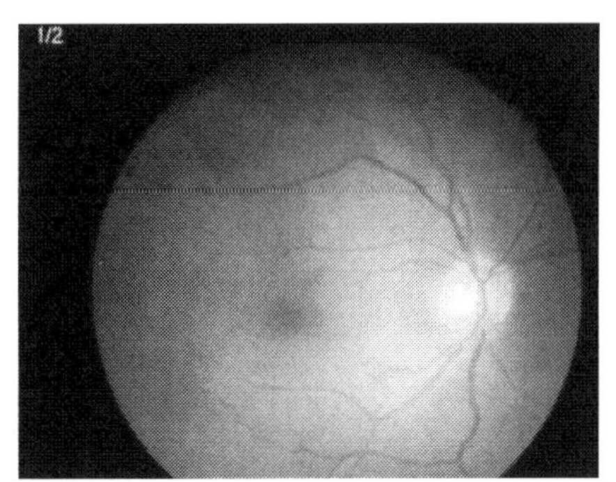

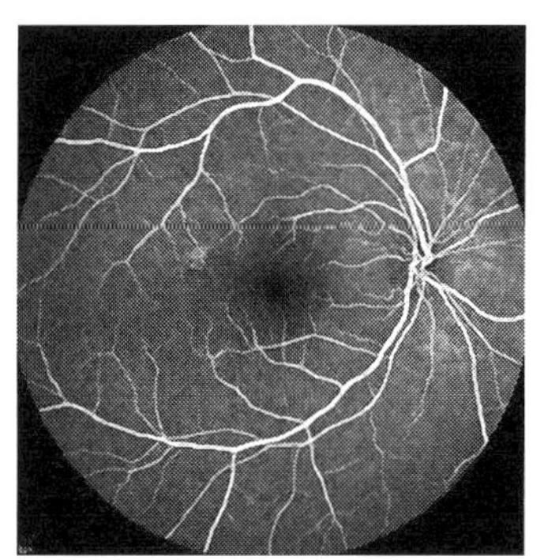

Photos: Retina of the eye and a Fluorescein angiogram

Electrodiagnostic Testing

Electrodiagnostic testing is not part of a routine eye examination, but is included here because it is used in cases where there is suspicion of a disease process based on the findings of the routine eye examination. The technology for these specialized tests are not found in every doctor's office. Testing is most likely to be found at a specialist's office or a referral center. It requires someone who is trained to administer the test and someone who is knowledgeable in interpreting the results.

Each of these electrodiagnostic tests are used to specifically evaluate different parts of the visual system. The tests are objective, meaning no responses are required on the part of the patient. These are measurements of the neurological electrical activity of the various cells of the visual system.

Electrodiagnostic testing is used to:

- Determine the cause of unexplained loss of visual acuity;
- Establish a diagnosis;
- Monitor the progression of a disease; and
- Test the visual acuity and visual function of a patient that is unable to respond.

1. Visual Evoked Potential (VEP)

   Visually evoked potential is also referred to as visual evoked response (VER) and visual evoked cortical potential (VECP). This electrodiagnostic test is measuring the electrical responses to light and pattern stimuli by the brain. VEP is used when the retina appears normal, but there is an unexplained decrease in vision. The visual cortex of the brain and the optic nerve, connecting the eye to the brain, need to be evaluated as the potential source of decreased visual acuity or visual function.

   The test is done by placing three electrodes on the scalp of the patient. Light or pattern stimuli are presented to the eye of the patient. The response of the brain is recorded by the instrument as electrical impulses. If a decrease of electrical activity is detected, a problem of the visual cortex of the brain or the optic nerve is suspected.

VEP is most often used for cases of;

- Unexplained decrease in visual acuity;
- Traumatic brain injury;
- Suspected multiple sclerosis (MS);
- Optic nerve disease: and
- Brain lesions along the visual pathway.(3)

It can also be used to measure visual acuity in patients that are unable to respond (infants and disabled adults).

2. Electroretinogram (ERG)

An electroretinogram is used to measure the electrical responses of the photoreceptors and other specialized ganglion cells of the retina. This test requires one electrode placed on the front of the eye and a second one placed on the skin. Light and pattern stimuli are presented to the patient, and the electrical response of the specialized cells of the retina are measured. Measurements can be taken for specific areas of the retina (multifocal ERG) or the retina as a whole. The test can even be modified to test specifically the rod or the cone photoreceptors. A decrease in the electrical response indicates a decrease in the function of the light responsive cells of the retina.

ERG is most often used in cases of:

- Unexplained decrease in visual acuity;

- Diagnosis of inherited retinal diseases, like retinitis pigmentosa, Leber's Congenital Amaurosis, choroideremia, x-linked retinoschisis, and other rod/cone dystrophies;
- Central nervous system disorders, with ocular involvement;
- Medical drug toxicity;
- Retinal vascular disease;
- Diabetic retinopathy; and
- Glaucoma.(4)

An ERG can often detect retinal eye disease before it becomes apparent.

3. Electrooculogram (EOG)

The electrooculogram is a test used to evaluate visual functioning at the level of the retinal pigment epithelium, which is an important support structure for the retina. Electrodes are placed on the skin around the eyes. The patient is asked to move their eyes back and forth between two light stimuli. First measurements are taken in the dark, then in the light. A decrease in electrical activity indicates a functional problem with the retinal pigment epithelium.

EOG is more specifically used for cases of:

- Bests' disease, in which the ERG is normal but the EOG will be depressed; and
- RPE dystrophies like Stargardt's Disease.(5)

References

1. Recommended Eye Examination Frequency for Pediatric Patients and Adults. American Optometric Association. Retrieved from **http://www.aoa.org/**]

2. Essential OCT, The Stratus OCT Primer Bressler, Neil M., MD, Ahmed, Iqbal Ike K., MD,Nguyen, Quan Dong, MD MSC, Shah, Namood, MD, Do, Diana V. MD, Hwang, Thomas,MD,Carl Zeiss Meditec AG Goeschwitzer Strasse, 2006'.

3. Visually Evoked Response (VER) or Potential (VEP). LKC Technologies, 2007-2015. Retrieved from **http://www.lkc.com/clinical/**

4. Electroretinogram (ERG). LKC Technologies, 2007-2015. Retrieved from **http://www.lkc.com/clinical/**

5. Electro-oculogram (EOG). LKC Technologies, 2007-2015. Retrieved from **http://www.lkc.com/clinical/**

6. Creel, Donnell J. The Electroretinogram and Electro-oculogram: Clinical applications. Webvision The Organization of the Retina and Visual System. Retrieved from **www.webvision.med.utah.edu**

CHAPTER 7

The Low Vision Evaluation

Those with low vision may feel the end of the road is the stronger glasses or the magnifier they picked up at the department store or flea market. More savvy shoppers may surf the internet looking for vision aids. Many of these purchases will be put aside because they just really don't help, are difficult to use, or impractical. Inexpensive aids may be of poor quality with distortions and aberrations, or may be too strong or not strong enough, which can cause eye strain. More sophisticated visual aids may require instruction for proper use.

Low vision means that new adjustments and adaptions must be made. There is no one magical vision aid that will do it all for the visually impaired. The average low vision patient has 3 to 4 vision aids to help with different visual tasks. Sorting out the best options and techniques is the job of the low vision practitioner. The benefit of the low vision evaluation is to gain an understanding of the disease process and associated vision loss, and to maximize visual acuity and visual function with the use of optical and non-optical aids.

The American Optometric Association outlines the goals of the low vision evaluation:

1. The low vision doctor will evaluate the whole system, medical and visual to help the patient determine what visual functions and capabilities they have left.

   "To assess ocular health and related medical health conditions and the impact of the disease or abnormal conditions on visual functioning."

2. Evaluate, set goals, and provide solutions to maximize remaining vision to help the patient adjust to a life with impaired vision.

   "To provide appropriate optometric rehabilitation intervention to improve the patient's special visual demands, needs, and adjustment to vision loss."

3. Counsel and educate the patient about their vision loss and the options available for treatment and rehabilitative services:

   "To counsel and educate patients regarding their visual impairment and ocular and systemic health status including recommendations for treatment, management, and future care."

4. Help the individual to coordinate comprehensive care and assistance with other therapists, specialists and counselors.

   "To provide appropriate referral for services that are outside the expertise of the optometric low vision clinician." (1)

The low vision doctor will help the patient determine what visual capabilities and functions they have left. The doctor will try to maximize the remaining capabilities and vision in order to maintain economic and social independence. Goals will be determined, like reading and other activities of daily living. An individual rehabilitation program should be established to determine which types of aids and technologies will help, and instruction and training in their use.

An informed patient has the potential to be a successful patient.

The Low Vision Evaluation

The low vision evaluation may repeat some of the prior testing you might have already experienced. The low vision practitioner, however, may be looking at a different aspect of that test, or in the case of a progressive disease, may be evaluating the updated results of that test.

A baseline must be established as a starting point. The best place to start is for you to bring in any eyeglasses that you have been using, any visual aids you might have picked up, and any materials, such as reading, hobbies, or work-related materials to help you and the doctor set goals as to what you would like to be able to accomplish. It is also helpful to have your eye doctor's records or a letter of findings to give the low vision practitioner an introduction, which leads to the first aspect of the low vision evaluation, the history.

History

Similar to a regular eye examination, the doctor will delve into your visual, medical, and medication history. The difference is that there will be questions regarding psychological, social, living, and work situations. The doctor will want to know how you are adapting and if you have a support system. He or she will also be listening for clues as to your level of acceptance and motivation.

The low vision doctor will look at any letters or records sent from the referring doctor as to previous testing and working diagnosis. The examiner will want to know if the disease process is stable or in the process of changing, and what is the prognosis. Presenting your current eye wear and vision aids will supplement the visual history. The clinician will want to know if you have experienced any recent changes in vision.

Medical history is also important. Since the visual system is an integral part of the whole body, health issues along with medications can affect the eyes. Be prepared to discuss health concerns and bring along with you a list of current medications.

The doctor will want to know where you are at in regards to acceptance, adjustment, and adaption. This is the psychosocial aspect of low vision care. How are you coping with the challenges? Are you able to maintain independence, like working and functioning on your own? Is there a support system available to you, and should any family or friends be included in the education and/or counseling process? Through the history interview process, the low vision clinician is not only looking at your visual impairment and medical health, but is also looking to get an insight into your emotional reaction to vision loss and attitude toward low vision services.

Task Analysis

Task analysis is how you and the low vision doctor determine what your needs are and to set goals. The discussion about tasks is to examine which activities of daily living (ADL) are hampered by the vision impairment, and need to be addressed in the rehabilitation process.

- What specifically do you have trouble seeing?
- problems seeing in the distance?
- problems seeing at near?
- problems with colors?
- problems with sunlight, interior lighting, or glare?
- problems with mobility or travel?
- difficulties performing work?
- difficulties performing household tasks?

The examiner also wants to know what you have already done to help yourself in these situations.

- Have magnifiers helped?
- Does large pint help?
- Do changes in lighting help?

– Do you wear sunglasses?

– Do you get help from others?

– What have you given up?

Through a comprehensive history and task analysis, you and the doctor have defined the difficulties and can begin to formulate goals.

Evaluation of Visual Function

Visual function is the sum of all the parts of the eye. A defect (disease or damage) of any part of the eye is considered an impairment. Some visual impairments have a greater, more devastating impact on vision than others.

Some aspects of the visual function evaluation may seem familiar from the routine eye examination. However, this time around, the examiner will be looking to evaluate visual capabilities as they may relate to activities of daily living, such as: reading, mobility, work, school, and watching television.

Visual Acuity

Visual acuity is tested first and foremost. It measures the patients' ability to see details. The low vision examiner will typically uses a different chart than the ones used during the routine examination. Low vision charts are designed with more lines of letters or numbers to better define visual capability. The low vision charts are usually free standing and can be moved forward a closer distance to the patient. These charts are high contrast, meaning that it is black letters or numbers on a white background. A more exact visual acuity test is important because it is used as the basis for determining magnification for both distance and near. The doctor is determining which eye is dominant and which eye can see better.

Near visual acuity will also be tested. The doctor is interested in where the patient holds their reading materials and their capability to read sentences or paragraphs. Reading a single letter on a chart is a measure of visual acuity, whereas reading sentences is a measure of visual function. The doctor will listen to whether or not the patient is reading accurately and the speed at which they are able to read.

Refraction

Refraction is the determination of the optimal eyeglass prescription. "Best corrected visual acuity" is the term used to indicate the best possible vision with the best eye glass prescription. Refraction can indicate a change in eyeglass prescription which can help the doctor determine where the patient is in the progression of their disease. Patients with cataracts can experience changes in refraction, month to month. A diabetic patient can experience changes in prescription, as determined by the refraction, day to day. It is during the refraction test that the doctor may begin to introduce modifications, such as stronger lenses and/or prisms. The magnification of glasses and other vision aids is initially determined by the visual acuity and refraction tests

Contrast Sensitivity

Contrast sensitivity testing is performed to measure visual function in the real world. The world is not high contrast black and white, but rather a gradient of shades. Contrast is how objects stand out from the background. Whereas visual acuity is based strictly on size and spacing, contrast sensitivity depends on light and reflection off object detail versus the background.

There are several different ways to test contrast sensitivity. Most tests consist of lines, letters, or numbers printed on a chart or sometimes on cards. Each line of numbers or letters is printed in a lighter shade than the line before it. Another type presents sets of lines that vary in thickness and distance between the lines. This variable separation between the lines is referred to as the spatial frequency. The greater the spatial frequency, the more detail, and therefore, more difficult for the eye to separate the lines from the background.

Photos:

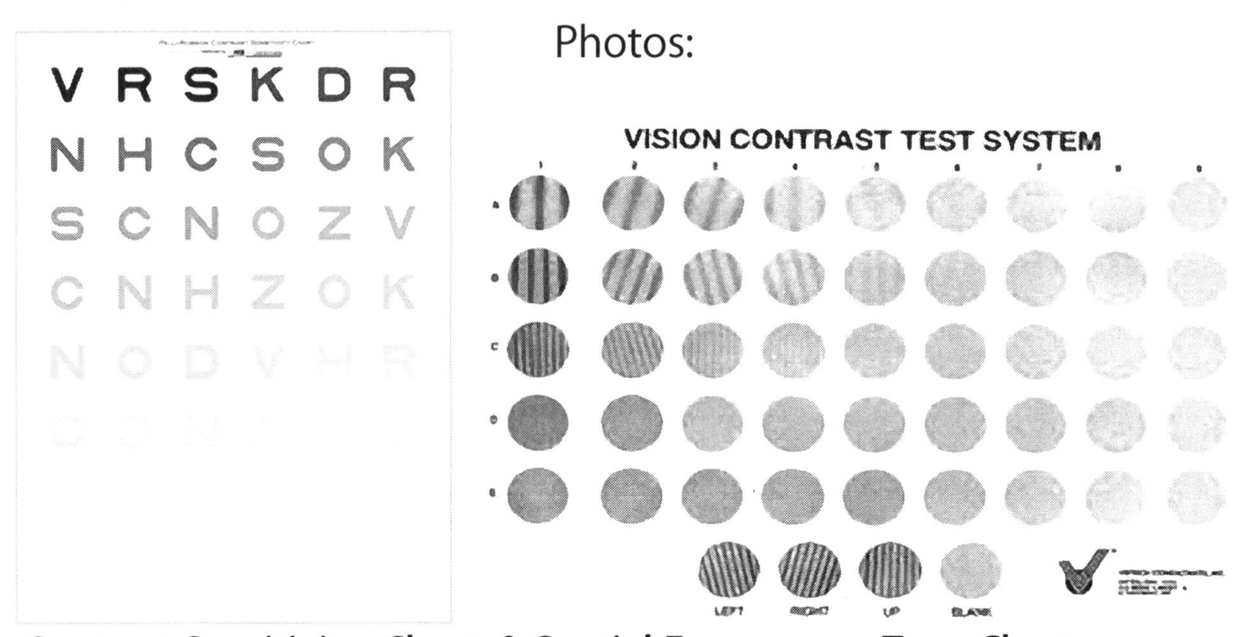

Contrast Sensitivity: Chart, & Spatial Frequency - Type Chart

Low contrast sensitivity indicates an overall depression in visual function, and makes it difficult for patients to see in low illumination (light) or to read materials of poor quality. Most patients with eye disease, have decreased or low contrast sensitivity. Measuring contrast sensitivity helps determine:

1. What light levels are needed for activities such as reading;
2. The need for enhanced contrast, important for the selection of optical aids; and
3. The patient needs enhanced magnification, more than might be atypically expected.

Glare

If a patient complains of glare, a doctor may choose to perform glare testing. Glare is the result of light scattering within the eye. Any opacities of the lens, cornea, or vitreous will result in glare. This will influence light levels, and the use of tints and filters.

Visual Field

Prior to the low vision evaluation, a visual field test using automated technology may have already been done as a part of the eye examination performed by the diagnosing doctor. The visual field test evaluates the sensitivity of the central and peripheral retina to identify blind spots. Visual field tests are often repeated to monitor changes in peripheral visual fields, and in the case of the low vision examination, it is used to determine where and how much damage the retina has sustained. Visual field analysis can reveal if a damaged area is totally lost (absolute) or just decreased in sensitivity (relative). When the rehabilitation process and any accompanied training begins, an understanding of the field of vision will help the therapist determine what can be accomplished and the appropriate program of therapy.

The Amsler Grid

The Amsler Grid test is frequently performed to determine blind spots or areas of distortion in the central 10 digress of vision. This central area of the macula is important because this is where our most sensitive visual acuity is located.

This test gives the patient a chance to describe other aspects of their vision. The 'Amsler' is a grid of horizontal and vertical lines. The patient should wear their near vision glasses, without magnifiers, and there should be good lighting. Covering one eye, the patient holds the Amsler grid 11 to 11 ¾ inches (28 to 30 cm) from their uncovered eye. A person with residual central vision will be able to focus on the central dot. Those with complete central loss will place the central blind area over the chart where two lines cross. Now observe:

1. How large is the blind area (how many blocks are obscured)? Each block, at 11 inches, represents one degree. The macular (central) area is 8 degrees horizontal by 6 degrees vertical.

2. If there is a central vision area, as in those patients with ring scotomas, how many blocks can be seen around the central dot?

3. Without moving the eye from the central dot (or where the lines

should cross in the obscured central area), are there any lines or blocks that appear to be missing? These would be scotomas.

4. Are there any lines that do not appear straight? Distortion may appear to be a single wavy line or entire areas where the blocks are not in straight lines. These would be defined as area of metamorphopsia.

This is a test of observation. Each eye is evaluated while the other eye is covered. Just as eye care professionals may use the Amsler grid as a tool to evaluate vision; it is also a good tool for patients to monitor their own vision. Changes in the scotomas or changes in distortion can be monitored. This observation can be helpful to the doctor when you return for your next evaluation. Any sudden changes in scotoma size or increase in distortion warrants an urgent examination.

Neurological Testing

Eye muscle movements are checked. This is done by holding the head still; while the eyes follow a moving target. The examiner is looking at how the eyes move, the alignment, how far they move, and for signs of nystagmus. The patient is to observe for areas of discomfort on movement or double vision.

Color Vision Evaluation

Color vision is routinely performed with Ishihara plates. These standardized color plates each have a matrix of colored dots with a number or shape hidden by utilizing colors hues commonly confused by those with color deficiencies. The Ishihara test determines hereditary color vision deficiencies in the red-green spectrums. A low vision doctor, if changes in color vision perception are suspected, may perform additional testing with the D-15 Dichotomous color test or Farnsworth color vision test. These tests employ colored caps. The patient is asked to line the caps up with the proceeding cap which is most similar in color. These tests will determine color vision deficiencies acquired through eye disease.

Photo:

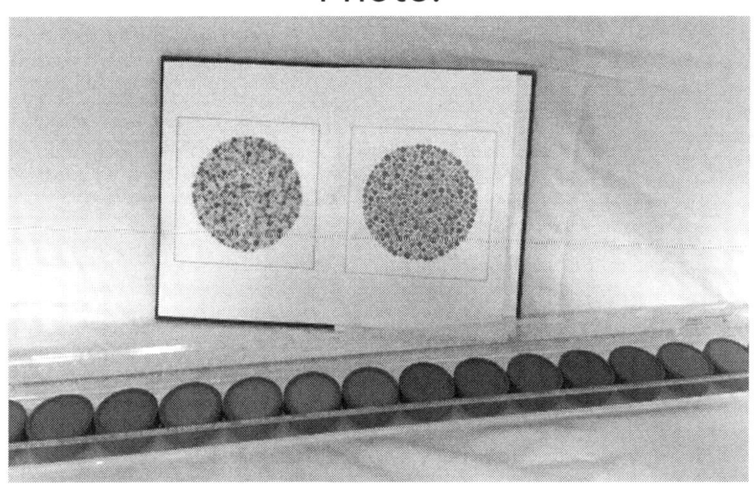

Ishihara color plates, and D-15 test

Conclusion

The low vision examination has given the examiner a baseline. Through the history, task analysis, and functional evaluation, the examiner establishes, with the patient's help, goals for selection of vision aids to help with activities of daily living, work, leisure activities, and/or school. This process will need to be repeated as life activities, needs, and the vision changes.

The next step is to learn how to effectively use new vision aid devices and techniques of adaption. This is called rehabilitation therapy.

Amsler Grid

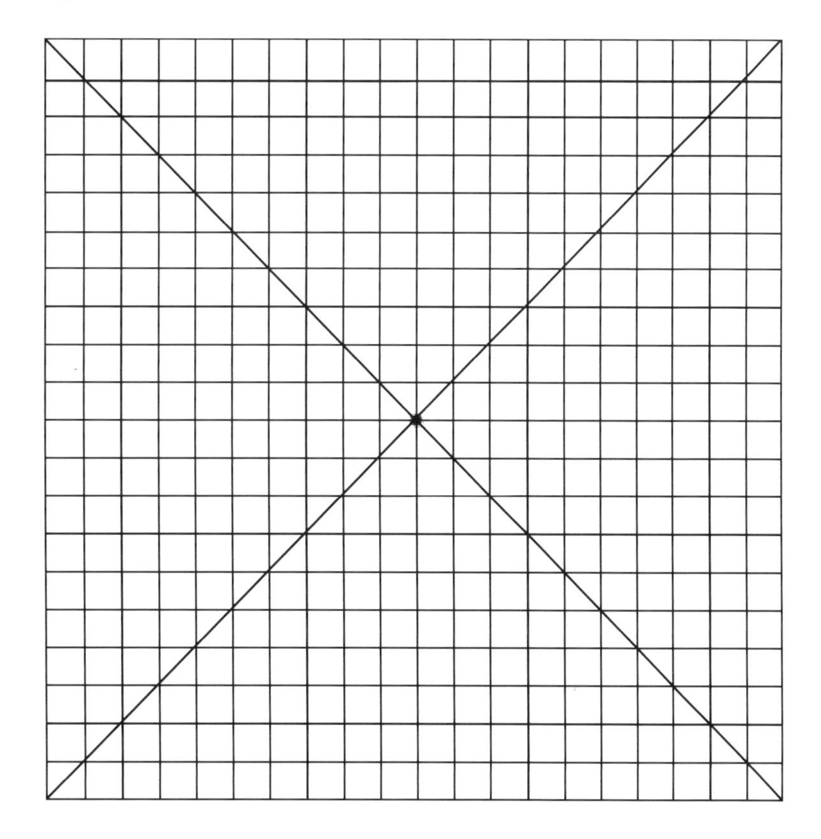

Cover one eye. Hold the chart 28 - 30 cm from your uncovered eye. This book is nearly 28 cm in length (11 inches).

Keep your eye focused on the center of the chart, and observe:

- Can you see all four corners and sides ?
- Are there any places where the lines of the grid are missing or blurred?
- Are there any places where the lines and squares are not straight?

Resources

1. Care of the Patient with Vision Impairment (Low Vision Rehabilitation. Optometric Clinical Practice Guideline. Retrieved from **www.aoa.org/documents/**

2. Faye, E. Clinical Low Vision. Boston: Little Brown, 1984

3. Faye E., Albert D. L., Freed B., Seidman K. R., Fischer M. The Lighthouse Ophthalmology Resident Training Manual, A New Look At Low Vision Care. New York: Lighthouse International. 2000.

4. Freeman P.B., Jose R. T. The Art and Practice of Low Vision. 2nd Edition. Boston Oxford Johannesburg Melbourne New Delhi Singapore. Butterworth-Heinemann. 2009.

CHAPTER 8

Types of Vision Loss

There are many ways in which vision is affected by the disease process. Many changes are typical for a disease, and commonly it is a combination of these changes that contribute to the loss of visual acuity and visual function. Acuity is the ability to see fine lines and forms as measured by the visual acuity charts used by your eye doctor. More elusive than visual acuity is the loss of visual function, which is not so easily measured. Interestingly, someone can have a good (measured) visual acuity, however may struggle to use their eyes in real life situations, where contrast is poor or lighting is too dim or bright. Conversely, someone can have a very poor (measured) visual acuity, however they still have good adaptive visual capability and can function quite well.

Vision loss can be described by any of the following terms independently, however there is frequently more than one factor that contributes to vision impairment.

Blur

Most familiar to us is the concept of blur. Blur describes an area of indistinct vision where lines and details are not seen as sharply and clearly. Blur can result in both a loss of visual acuity and a loss of visual function. It can be generalized as a term meaning an overall haziness, or it can just be an area of indistinct vision. . If the blur occurs in the central area of the eye (the macula), the experience can be devastating to visual acuity. A blurry area in the peripheral vision will not have as great an impact on visual acuity.

Many people experience a temporary blur, such as uncorrected refractive error (someone who needs eye glasses or an updated prescription) or transient, like having dry eyes. Blur can occur as a result of a systemic condition, such as uncontrolled blood sugar, migraines, or side effects of a medication. These conditions are temporary, and can be resolved.

Eye diseases are a primary cause of blur. Cataracts are the most common of eye anomalies to cause blurry vision. Fortunately, it is one of the eye problems that can be resolved with surgery. Retinal or optic nerve disease (which damages the sensitive photoreceptors of the retina), may result in permanent blur, which may not be resolved by surgery or medications.

Management of Blur

Those with unresolved blur will require assistive devices, such as magnifiers and telescopes, to compensate for the loss of the ability to see fine lines and details.

Loss of Contrast Sensitivity

Contrast is what makes an object stand out from the background. It is that difference in the reflected light from the objects versus the background. The visual system's ability to detect that difference is what is called contrast sensitivity. This is a more elusive part of our visual system's capability that is difficult to describe and can be difficult to measure.

The eye doctor can measure visual acuity using a visual acuity chart. The chart has the highest form of contrast, that is, with black letters on a white surface. However, this may not, reflect (no pun intended) how you see in the 'real' world, where the contrast between objects is not in black and white and light levels vary. When measured, the higher your contrast sensitivity, the lower the amount of light is needed for you to see objects. A person with significant low contrast sensitivity will see things as washed out or pale. Having a vision impairment does not necessarily mean there is loss of contrast sensitivity. Having said that, the reality is that most people who are visually impaired do have some reduced contrast sensitivity and do not realize their impairment.

An individual's contrast sensitivity is affected, not only by varying light levels, but also by the capability to see detail (visual acuity). Those visual impairments that result in blur can cause loss of contrast because of the inability to see edges and demarcation lines, therefore it is difficult to separate an object from the background.

Low contest sensitivity can have a detrimental effect on visual function. It can result in an inability to adapt to a change in light levels. Dim light situations have the least contrast, making it difficult to navigate in the environment. Walking downstairs or stepping off a curb in a dimly lit situation can be difficult. Reading material, such as the newspaper, in which there is not a high contrast of black on white, but instead a grey print on yellowish paper, or colored printing on a colored background, can be difficult to read.

Management of Contrast Sensitivity

Those individuals with low contrast sensitivity will benefit by:

1. Increased Light Levels. Optimize room and task lighting.

2. Electronic Technology. The best option is magnifiers that are illuminated. Even more helpful are those whose illumination levels can be controlled and give users the option to control print vs. background modes to increase contrast.

3. Eyeglass Tints. Certain eyeglass tints are optimal for enhancing contrast. See 'Light, Lenses, and the Eye'.

4. High Contrast Ink Pens. Pens that write with a broad, high contrast (black) ink optimize handwritten notes. Examples are felt tip markers and gel pens.

Light Sensitivity and Glare

Light levels for optimal visual performance vary by the eye condition and individual preferences. While some visual conditions benefit with an increase in light levels, other eye disease result in greater light sensitivity. Because of the way light sensitive neurons in our visual system are wired, those with retinal diseases may find the sunshine or bright lights exceedingly bright and have difficulty adapting, and in turn experience light sensitivity (photophobia). Those with Stargardt's disease, achromatopsia, or albinism will find increasing light levels uncomfortable.

Glare is another component that contributes to light sensitivity and loss of contrast sensitivity. Those with vision impairments may find high light levels difficult due to the glare. Glare can originate outside the eye, or be created within the eye itself. Glare occurs when a light source or object that reflects light, is bright enough to overpower the capability to see surrounding objects. The average, normal-sighted person experiences glare off reflective surfaces, like water, or driving into the late afternoon sun. Those with light sensitivity will be more sensitive to, and disabled by, external glare.

The other way glare can impact vision is by internal reflections within the visual system. Light entering a normal healthy eye has a clear path through the eye to the light sensing cells at the back of the eye. Any process that infringes on the clarity of the parts of the eye can cause scatter, meaning the light will not be crisply focused to the back of the eye, but will instead bounce around, creating the phenomenon of internal glare. Damage to the cornea, lens cataracts, and vitreous floaters, can contribute to internal glare.

Management of Light Sensitivity and Glare

Light sensitivity and problems with glare needs to be addressed with your eye care professional. Light and glare sensitivity are difficult to measure in the exam room. Although those with certain eye impairments are known to have increased susceptibility to light sensitivity and glare.

1. Tints, Filters, Polarization, and Anti-reflective Coatings. Those that experience light sensitivity and glare will benefit from tints, filters, polarization, and anti-reflective coatings on the lenses of their eyeglasses. Consider tints that decrease light transmission to the eye for those with light sensitivity, like shades of grey. Glare is reduced by cutting out UV and blue light by a yellow or amber tint which absorbs blue light.(1) Sunglasses that are photochromic (change tint based on light exposure), are helpful to those with problems of light adaption. Polarization, combined with a tint, reduces the glare reflected off of horizontal surfaces. Anti-reflective coatings on lenses also reduce external glare and reflections off the lenses.

2. Hats with brims and visors. Headwear is useful to reduce light entering from above and help to reduce glare that causes discomfort. Sunglasses with tinted side shields help to reduce light which enters from the sides.

Visual Field Loss and Scotomas

The visual field is the entire area of vision which includes the central macula and the areas of vision to the sides, and up and down. The visual fields of both eyes overlap to give us a 'panoramic' view of the world (a total of about 190 degrees horizontally, for those people with normal binocular visual field!). Although these peripheral areas of vision are not as sensitive to the detail of line and form as the central macular area, our peripheral areas are sensitive to light and motion. These areas of vision help us to orient ourselves in our environment and enable us to move around efficiently. Loss of central vision means a loss of visual acuity; while the loss of peripheral vision impacts our orientation and mobility capabilities.

Scotomas are blind spots or areas of depressed vision. The impact of a blind spot is determined by location, size, depth, and whether it is in one eye or both. Scotomas occur where there is retinal cell death. Retinal cell death occurs either through the disease's degenerative process or by damage sustained because of bleeding, inflammation, trauma, or toxicity of medications.(2)

Location and Size of Visual Field Loss

Central scotomas are the most devastating to visual acuity. This central macular area is the area of most dense light sensitive neurons (cones) that give the most detailed visual information. This is the area devastated in age-related macular degeneration and the juvenile form, Stargardt's disease. Loss of central vision results in difficulty with reading (print disabled) and facial recognition. Although visual acuity is low, visual function can be maintained. Those with central loss can still have their peripheral vision to maintain good mobility and can learn to use eccentric fixation.

Ring scotomas are often the precursors to central vision loss. The blind spots occur around the macular area, either as spots or as a confluent ring. At this stage, visual acuity may still be good, but there may be some loss of function. An example would be reading, because of blind spots on the right side of the maculae. (We read left to right, information is initially processed right of the macula). Face recognition or reading signs is difficult, because areas may not be seen in totality due to the ring scotoma.

Peripheral field loss refers to the area outside the macula; it is the rest of the visual area. The areas of loss vision can be a section, entire hemispheres, or localized areas.

Sections of field losses are large areas of vision loss due to damage or disease. They will often leave a patient with good visual acuity if the central area is not involved. Overall visual function may be good if the lost visual field of one eye is not matched by an equal one in the other eye. That is, one eye's loss visual field is normally compensated for by the still healthy visual field of the other eye, when both eyes are open. Glaucoma and optic neuritis are examples of diseases in which large sections of arcuate scotomas may extend from the peripheral field of the retina to the optic nerve. If this occurs in just one eye, vision may only be affected by an inability to see in the very far peripheral area on one side. The good eye sees all the rest, and compensates for the bad eye. But if both eyes have large superior arcuate scotomas, the glaucoma patient, with this type of matching visual field loss, will become aware of the missing areas of vision. In this example, it would be in the lower field (going downstairs would be difficult.)

Hemispheric scotomas occur to an entire one quarter or one half of the visual field. Often they occur secondary to vascular events (ex: strokes) or tumors within the brain (ex: pituitary tumors). The macula may be spared, in which case, good visual acuity can be maintained. If the macula is also affected, there will be a loss of visual acuity. The same rule applies to these very large areas of vision loss; if it is just one eye, it is not as devastating a loss than if both eyes are affected.

Large area of vision loss can greatly affect functioning. These blind areas can make it difficult to navigate. Objects and architecture on the side may not be seen and can result in collisions.

Retinitis pigmentosa is one of the most dramatic of diseases of visual field loss. Retinitis pigmentosa is a degenerative disease which can affect large areas of retina, often wiping out the entire peripheral visual field. The end stages of retinitis pigmentosa result in a total loss of peripheral vision and a phenomenon of keyhole vision (or tunnel vision). In this case, the field of vision is a very small 10 to 20 degrees.

Depth of Visual Field Loss

Depth refers to the degree of visual field loss. There can be a complete loss of light sensitivity, referred to as absolute, meaning no vision in that area. The field loss which is partial, also known as relative, means the area of visual field is less sensitive relative to the surrounding retina. An example is a person who has glaucoma and visual field loss on the far periphery. They find themselves bumping into door jams or furniture, because they absolutely have no vision on that side. A person with diabetes may only experience decreased or 'washed out' vision in the peripheral retina relative to the rest of their vision. Those with relative visual field defects benefit from increased illumination and/or contrast.

Tools and Techniques of Field Enhancement

Those who have lost central macular vision benefit from eccentric fixation training. Eccentric fixation is a technique in which another part of the retina is used for 'seeing.' This technique can be trained, but often it is learned by self discovery. Although this new area does not see as well as the macula once did, adaptive technology like glasses and magnifiers can help visual function.

Those who have large scotomas, where there are large sections of vision loss, benefit from the use of field enhancers. A Fresnel prism is a thin plastic film, placed on the eyeglasses, in the area of the lost visual field. It is composed of little rows of prisms that shift the image from the non-seeing area toward the central vision area, to make the wearer aware of objects in that field without a lot of eye movement. It takes practice to adapt to using the Fresnel prism effectively. Objects seen through a Fresnel prism may not be sharp and clear, but the user's visual field is enhanced for orientation and object localization

A technique taught to those with large or constricted visual field loss is the technique of scanning. Scanning is a systematic approach to help assess the environment and localize objects. It is a skill that requires training and practice.

Those who have lost most of their visual field to a disease such as retinitis pigmentosa, benefit from field expanders, like high minus lenses and reverse telescopes. These devices will give a wider field of view, by minification. (Minification is the opposite of magnification. It makes objects appear smaller.) Therefore, good for localizing the surrounding environment; however at the cost of losing details. Surrounding objects will also appear farther away. These field expanders are not used constantly, but are used briefly in a stationary position for spotting and orienting.

Those with large visual field losses and constricted visual fields have trouble reading and tracking along lines of print. When we read, our vision outside the central vision area orients us to where we are on the page and is useful for helping us track back to the next line of print. Typoscopes are black masks that have long slots cut out, that are placed over a line of print. It masks the rest of the page to highlight the line of print to be read. These serve as a guide for the reader. There are also typoscopes specifically designed to fill out personal checks.

Distortion

Most commonly this is a phenomenon experienced in the central vision area called the macula, but can occur anywhere in the visual field. Imagine the light sensitive photoreceptor cells standing up straight like soldiers, elbow to elbow, orderly in rows. Should these photoreceptors somehow become disrupted, by fluids or waste toxins moving in between them, they are no longer orderly, but are in a bit of disarray. The brain perceives this disarray as distortion. Lines on the road may not appear straight, edges of walls may appear to lean, and letters of words appear jumbled up.

Fluid underneath or within the macula or retina push the

photoreceptors out of alignment. This is commonly called edema. Edema can occur as a consequence of diabetes, retinal vein occlusions, post-surgery, retinal detachments, and 'wet' age-related macular degeneration.

Drusen are hard, yellowish retractile deposits within the retina. Their greatest impact is when they are located in the macula. They are formed as a byproduct of cell metabolism that have not been recycled by the degenerating cells. These drusen can be toxic. These deposits can cause disruption of the orderly alignment of the photoreceptors. They are commonly found in dry macular degeneration, Stargardt's disease, and diabetic retinopathy.

Management of Distortion

There is no compensatory technique or technology to elevate distortion. Resolution of the underlying edema, by medical treatment can help resolve some cases of distortion.

Nystagmus

Nystagmus refers to the rhythmic, involuntary movement of the eyes resulting in decreased vision. The eyes may appear to 'jiggle.' The term used for 'jiggling' of the eyes is oscillopsia. This movement does not permit fixation for observation of a detail, therefore a detail appears blurred.

The movement varies by direction, for example, side to side, up and down, or even in a circular motion.(3) The amount of movement can also vary by magnitude, that is, by size of the movement, speed, and frequency of movement. These variables of magnitude can be exacerbated by fatigue, excitement, or stress.

Nystagmus can be congenital (born with), or infantile (manifests in the first two years of life), or acquired later in life. Nystagmus, most commonly, is the result of a vision impairment rather than being the primary cause of the impairment, and ultimately does add to the disability.

Children with nystagmus may have an associated neurological disorder or vision impairment such as albinism, achromatopsia, Leber's Congenital Amaurosis and other macular anomalies, optic nerve anomalies, or congenital opacities of the cornea or cataracts.(4) Those who have congenital nystagmus are unaware of the constant eye movement.

The types acquired by adults are commonly associated with problems of the vestibular apparatus (inner ear), brain lesions, nerve trauma, drug interaction, drug toxicity, or neurological disease. Nystagmus developed later in life can be devastating to vision. A person who develops nystagmus later in life will be aware of the movement and may experience nausea or disorientation.(5)

Because of the link between the vestibular system of the ear and eye movements, diseases such as Meniere's Disease can cause a particular type of nystagmus called jerk nystagmus. Jerk nystagmus is a slow movement of the eye in one direction, followed by a rapid movement back in the opposite direction.

Some people, predominantly those with congenital nystagmus, are able to find a null point, which is a gaze in a particular direction or a particular distance, usually near, in which the 'jiggling' subsides. At the null point, the vision is the best. A person who finds a null point may develop a head turn or a tilt of the head to align their gaze to the null point for better vision.

Management of Nystagmus

Treatment for nystagmus depends on the underlying cause. Optical, surgical, and medical treatments are still a matter of research. Finding the null point and utilizing it to dampen the oscillopsia, can improve visual acuity.

1. Optical. Low vision specialists determine the null point location. Spectacle lenses are designed that not only incorporate the optimal prescription, but also have prisms ground in to the lens. Prisms stabilize the eye movement by utilizing the null point. The prisms deflect the image onto the retina of the wearer at the determined null point. Essentially the lenses are doing the work of a head turn or tilt, so the wearer can look straight ahead and maintain a normal head position.

2. Contact Lenses. Contact lenses have been used by a few with nystagmus, who need glasses to achieve their best vision. They can do better with contact lenses, because the contacts move with the eyes. Others have suggested that the sensation of a rigid gas permeable contact lens, which touches the upper eye lid, gives a kind of biofeedback, making the wearer aware of eye movement, and as a result the movement is dampened.(6)

3. Surgery and Medical Treatment. Surgery is done on the eye muscles to either tighten or loosen them to align the eye to the null point. This is to dampen the motion, reduce the need for

head turns and tilts, and ideally optimize vision. Unfortunately, it can result in a loss of some normal range of eye movement.

Medications have also been researched as a means of dampening the oscillopsia.(7) Botulinum Neurotoxin A is an injection that has had some success, for those with acquired nystagmus, to improve visual function.(8)

Color Vision Anomalies

Color deficiencies occur as a congenital anomaly or are acquired as part of a disease process. The term color blind is a term frequently used to describe a common congenital color deficiency that affects 8 to 10 percent of the population, predominantly male. This relatively common form of color vision anomaly is really better termed a as color deficiency or partial color vision. It is not that they don't see color; it is that they are lacking the photo-pigment that is sensitive to certain wavelengths of light. Most frequently the deficiency is in the red-green wavelengths. This means that hues of red and green look similar and are confused. For example, an inability to detect red means that purple, which is a combination of blue and red, will appear blue to a person with a red deficiency, because they are not sensitive to the red even when combined with blue. An even rarer anomaly is a color deficiency in the blue-yellow range. These vision anomalies, which are congenital, affect both eyes equally, and are stable, meaning it is not part of a disease process, and will not get worse.(9)

Another type of congenital color anomaly is achromatopsia,

also known as rod monochromacy. This congenital condition is a deficiency of all 3 photo-pigments: red, green, and blue. The deficiency of achromatopsia can have varying degrees of severity. The most severe being color blind, that is, lacking in color perception. Those with this deficiency will be extremely light sensitive, have decreased visual acuity, and nystagmus.(10) They benefit from protective eyewear and filters.

Acquired color deficiencies differ from congenital, in that they occur after birth and are associated with a disease process. Therefore are not stable, and may affect one eye more than the other. Changes in color sensitivity are usually accompanied by a decrease in visual acuity. Hereditary eye diseases such as Best's Vitelliform Dystrophy, Stargardt's Disease (juvenile macular degeneration), and retinitis pigmentosa can manifest color sensitivity changes as the disease progresses.

Adult onset diseases such as diabetes, glaucoma, and cataracts can affect color vision. Interestingly, lens cataracts act as a yellow filter that can influence color perception. Unlike other disease processes, where the color sensitive cells are damaged or destroyed, surgical removal of the lens with cataracts solves the color problem.

Optic nerve diseases, such as optic atrophy or optic neuritis, can affect color perception. The optic nerve is the bundle of nerves, sort of like a cable, that extends from the retina of the eye to the visual area of the brain, carrying nerve impulses of light and form perception. An inflammation of the nerve and myelin sheath covering the optic nerve is called optic neuritis. The result is a decrease in visual acuity and a perception of colors as pale and washed out. Those with multiple sclerosis, autoimmune diseases, and either bacterial or viral infections can develop optic nerve inflammation. Once the inflammation is resolved, vision can return to normal or near normal.

Optic nerve atrophy is a process in which the nerves of the optic nerve are dying. This can also result in decreased visual acuity, scotomas and visual field loss, and loss of color perception. Diseases that affect the blood flow to the eye and optic nerve, such as strokes, hypertension, exposure to toxins (alcohol abuse), and trauma can cause optic nerve atrophy.

Management of Color Deficiencies

There is no treatment for congenital forms of color deficiency. Acquired forms of color deficiency are managed by treatment of the underlying condition. Color deficiencies that are acquired because of a disease process will most likely not be resolved if there is permanent neurological damage.

Colored eyeglass filters and colored contact lenses can be used to help with color discrimination. This does not create color vision for the wearer, but does help the user distinguish color by differences in brightness or darkness of colors which are normally confused. In this way, the filter enhances the differences of colors that look similar. Use of filters is dependent on the task, and what colors need to be differentiated. Eye care specialists prescribe these specialty lenses and provide counseling and training as to their use.

"Is there an app for that?" Of course there is. There are several apps that use the camera of your mobile device to identify colors.

Type 'color identifier' into the app store search bar. This has been available to the blind community by way of hand-held assistive technology that speaks colors. There is also computer software designed to help with color determination for those professionals who need help identifying colors for things like web design. Search for color recognition software.

Double Vision

Double vision can be monocular or binocular. Monocular double vision presents as two images seen with just one eye open. Cover one eye, then the other. If the doubling of the image is still present with just one eye open, it is monocular diplopia. The causes of monocular double vision can be as mundane as uncorrected astigmatism, which can be corrected by eyeglasses, or as part of a disease process in which there is a disruption of the cornea, such as keratoconus, scarring of the cornea, or disruption of the lens, such as cataracts or trauma.

Binocular double vision occurs only when both eyes are open, and the images from each eye are not aligned. Normally the images of both eyes are fused together. When the visual system developed before birth, the nerves and muscles of the eyes were 'yoked'. This pairing of the nerves and muscles assures alignment of the point of fixation and movement of the eyes so they are equal, to maintain a single image. A process that damages, impedes, or destroys the nerves or muscles will disrupt the 'yoke' and double vision can occur. (The analogy refers to a team of oxen that have a yoke, so they move together in the same direction, at the same speed.)

Double vision can occur due to a disturbance along the visual pathway of the optic nerve, or in the visual cortex of the brain. It can cause one wayward eye or two. The double vision may occur when looking only in a particular direction or at a particular distance. Images may be side by side, up and down, or some other angle with a tilt. The distance between the two images may be large or appear as a slight ghosting of overlapping images. The double vision may be transient, (lasting for brief periods), episodic with resolution varying by the course of the underlying disease, or permanent.

Causes can be due to a neurological disorder such as myasthenia gravis, or neuromuscular disorders such as thyroid disease. Disorders of these types affect the nerves and/or the muscles that control eye movement by causing a partial paralysis (paresis) or full paralysis of the nerve or muscle. Vascular diseases such as diabetes and high blood pressure or vascular events such as stroke, similarly affect the function of the nerves and muscles of the eyes. Space occupying lesions such as tumors and pituitary adenomas can affect nerve and muscle function. Trauma to the head, face and orbital cavity of the eye can damage nerves or trap and damage muscles of the eye.

Management of Double Vision

Treatment depends on the underlying cause. Double vision will often resolve if the nerves and muscles are not permanently damaged.

Permanent diplopia can be managed with prisms ground into

the lenses of the eyeglasses. Prisms are not visible to someone observing the eyeglasses. It is a technique of making an area of the lens a little thicker, to bend the light rays, and therefore the image, to help the individual to fuse two images into one. The amount of prism varies by the amount of the deviation of the eyes. The measurement is very specific and needs to be done by a qualified professional.

References:

1. Ludt, Richard, Three types of Glare: Low Vision O+M Assessment and Remediation, Review, Rehabilitation and Education for Blindness and Vision Impairment. Volume 29 No. 3, Fall 1997, pg 109.
2. Michaels, David D., Visual Optics and Refraction A Clinical approach, Third Edition, The C.V. Mosby Company, pg, 555-556.
3. Nystagmus. Retrieved from **www.aoa.org** Home > Patients and Public > View All Resources > Glossary of all Eye and Vision Conditions > Nystagmus
4. Rosenbloom, Alfred A., Morgan, Meredith W., Principles and Practices of Pediatric Optometry, , J.B. Lippincott Company, pg 343-344.
5. Dickenson, Christine. Low Vision, Principles and Practice. Butterworth-Heineman. 2002, pg 210.
6. Nowakowski, Rodney W. Primary Low Vision Care. Appleton and Lange. pg 326.
7. Stahl, JS, Plant, GT, Leigh, J. Medical treatment of nystagmus and its visual consequences. J R Soc of Med. May 2002, 96(6). 235-237.
8. Repka, MX, Savino, PJ, Reinecke, RD. Treatment of acquired nystagmus with Botulinum neurotoxin A. Arch of Ophthalmol. 1994, 112(10):1320-1324.

9. Day, Nigel W., Hart Jr., William M., Color Vision (Chapter 22), Adler's Physiology of the Eye , Clinical Application, 8th ed., pg 579.

10. Achromatopsia. American Association for Pediatric Ophthalmology and Strabismus. Retrieved from **www.aapos.org**/..update 03/2015.

CHAPTER 9

Interesting (Not Totally Understood) Phenomenon

There are several unique visual experiences that some people diagnosed with progressive, degenerative eye diseases experience that are not a cause of the disease process, but are a transient experience as a result of the disease process and loss of vision. They are:

1. Fluctuating Vision
2. Photopsias
3. Visual Hallucinations: Charles Bonnet Syndrome.

Not everyone experiences these events, but for those who do, it can be scary, bewildering, disturbing, annoying, or even outright bizarre. Though it is impossible to "prepare" for these unique events, it is helpful to know and understand that it has happened to others with similar visual impairments.

Fluctuating Vision

Fluctuating vision can be described as having good or bad vision days, or noticing the changes in quality of vision between the morning and the evening. These experiences are not caused by the environmental (good light vs. poor light), but rather are physiological in nature.

These fluctuations in vision are biologically related. Some causes are understood by the medical community, others are not. For example, diabetics come to understand that their blood sugar level impacts not only how they feel overall, but a blood sugar that is off kilter effects their vision. Those with macular edema secondary to age-related macular degeneration (ARMD), will experience fluctuations with poorer vision upon awakening in the morning.(1) Both those with ARMD and diabetes experience vision fluctuation related to tissue fluid changes. But the complete mechanism for why vision fluctuates is a matter of research.

Individuals with retinitis pigmentosa, a progressive degenerative disease of the retina, can also experience fluctuations in vision. The medical community does not fully understood why this occurs .(2)

For people with nystagmus, a condition where eyes make repetitive and uncontrolled movements, their vision fluctuations are related to changes in the rate of eye movement, and is often associated with stress and fatigue.

Additionally, diseases or surgical procedures that affect the cornea can impact vision. This includes Fuchs Dystrophy (a progressive disease of the cornea), dry eyes, and commonly after refractive corrective surgery (LASIK). It is the transient changes to the corneal tissue that results in fluctuations of vision.

Physiological changes in vision cannot always be attributed to the disease process, but nay be caused by medications. A few very commonly prescribed medications can (not always) cause blurring of vision. These include: Tamoxifen, isotretinoin, Gileyma, steroids, erectile dysfunction medications, osteoporosis treatments and some anti-anxiety drugs.

The best thing to do is to monitor when vision fluctuations occur. This will allow you to work with the low vision doctor to determine if these experiences are a part of the disease process or a side effect of the medication.

Photopsia

This phenomenon varies from a flash of light to moving patterns of light. These lights appear randomly with no other visual associations. It can occur in one eye or both eyes. They have been seen by those with retinitis pigmentosa (2), age-related macular degeneration, and Stargardt's Disease.

Photopsia should be differentiated from light flashes associated with retinal detachment or traction on the retina. These are both active processes that can be a sign of potential vision loss. Photopic visual experiences, are thought to be residual neurological activity, as they occur in the area of retina which is already damaged. This would be analogous to the phantom pain experienced by those who have lost a limb. (3)

Visual Hallucinations: Charles Bonnet Syndrome

Charles Bonnet was an eighteenth century naturalist who was the first to describe visual hallucinations experienced by his grandfather, who was of 'clear mind' and visually impaired by cataracts. An individual receives the diagnosis of having Charles Bonnet Syndrome when they have vision loss, and no mental or psychological disorders, yet they experience very distinct, well-formed hallucinations.

Individuals with Charles Bonnet Syndrome describe seeing detailed images of people, animals, or complete scenes with movement. Sometimes these images merge into the surrounding environment, or the scene may change and become quite bizarre. The hallucination may be of people familiar to the viewer or they may be strangers. The scene may be commonplace or like a fairy tale.

Most importantly, the individual is well aware that the images are not real, and that is what separates the diagnosis of Charles Bonnet Syndrome from hallucinations experienced by those with psychiatric, cognitive, or medication/drug-related episodes.

To be diagnosed, a person must meet the following three criteria:

1. Vision loss;
2. Clearly formed, often recurrent hallucinations; and
3. Those that experience hallucinations are aware that they are not real.

Visual hallucinations can occur at any age and with any type of vision impairment, and are thought to occur in 10 - 35 percent of people with vision loss.(4) Many people who have these visual hallucinations, especially the elderly who are most often affected by age related macular degeneration, cataracts, or diabetic retinopathy, and live alone, may think they are going crazy. They typically will not report these symptoms to family and doctors for fear they will be placed in a mental institution, People who see these visual hallucinations. typically are socially isolated and lack stimulation.(4)

These Charles Bonnet Syndrome hallucinations have been called phantom vision, comparing it to the phantom pain experienced by those with a lost limb. This indicates these hallucinations are generated from visual memory and not from a psychotic break.

While there is no medical treatment, the visual hallucinations will subside over time. Social interaction, a change in environment, and mental stimulation can keep the mind busy and will help to decrease the symptoms.

In 2009, Oliver Sacks gave a TED Talk titled: "What hallucination reveals about our minds." He specifically discusses Charles Bonnet Syndrome. If you have internet access, this is a very interesting lecture!

References

1. Paques, Michael P., Nassani, Pascale, Sahel, Jose A., Gaudric, Alain, Bergman, Jean-Francois, Azancot, Suzanne, Levy, Bernard I., Vicaut, Eric. Circadian Fluctuations of Macular Edema in Patients with Morning Vision Blurring: Correlation with Arterial Pressure and Effect of Light

Deprivation. Inv Oph&Vis Sci. Dec. 2005.

2. Bittner,Ava K., OD,1 Edwards, Lori,, MPH, and George, Maureen, PhD. 3 Coping strategies to manage stress related to vision loss and fluctuations in retinitis pigmentosa. Optometry. 2010 Sep; 81(9): 461–468. **www.ncbi.nlm.nih.gov/**...
3. Schultz, G. Melzack, R., Visual hallucinations and mental state - a study of 14 Charles Bonnet hallucinations. J New Ment Disease 181: 1993, 639-643.
4. Jackson, M.L., MD and Ferencz, Joseph MD PhD Charles Bonnet syndrome: visual loss and hallucinations. CMAJ. 2009 Aug 4; 181(3-4): 175–176.
5. Menon GJ1, Rahman I, Menon SJ, Dutton GN. Complex visual hallucinations in the visually impaired: the Charles Bonnet Syndrome. Surv Ophthalmol. 2003 Jan-Feb;48(1):58-72
6. Murphy, C. When Seeing Isn't Believing: Charles Bonnet Syndrome. (August 9, 2012) *Scientific American*. Retrieved on September 5, 2012 from **http://www.scientificamerican.com/**.

CHAPTER 10

The Eye Disease and Its Impact on Vision

Any disease process that interferes with the integrity of the eye has the potential to cause vision loss. The eye is composed of specialized tissues in precise alignment resulting in the miraculous function of allowing us to see. This amazing structure is set on a stalk-like extension called the optic nerve that is integrated into the brain. The eye is indeed 'brain tissue' whose nerve endings are specialized for the detection of light, movement, color, and details of line and form. The brain is able to utilize this information to not only biochemically detect the light and forms, but also render an interpretation of what is seen, which is called perception.

Many times I have heard people say they could do without hearing, taste, touch, a limb, or some other body part, but could never do without sight. Indeed, it is our window to the world. From the time we wake in the morning to look at the clock, until we turn out the light at night, our vision guides us through our daily activities. So much so, that we take this amazing gift of sight for granted, until it no longer functions perfectly. It is a sighted world. That is why vision loss can be so devastating to those who are afflicted.

Loss of vision can affect anyone at any age. There are hundreds of diseases that can affect our eyes, either through heredity or acquired throughout our lives. There are those diseases that are more common than others. Most eye diseases are acquired throughout life, and are associated with age and influenced by health and environmental factors. Within this category of age-related diseases are those that are the proverbial time bombs; hereditary diseases that predispose us in our senior years to vision loss. This is the risk of eye disease indicated by a family history of the disease.

The second half of this chapter touches on the hereditary disorders that are either present at birth or a disease that reveals itself in the first few decades of life, and are more commonly associated with vision loss in the younger population.

The first half, I will discuss those diseases that are the most commonly seen in the doctor's office, and a few not so common, that rob so many of us of our vision.

Age-Related Macular Degeneration (ARMD)

ARMD is a disease of the central vision area (called the macula).. It can affect patients as early as their 40s, but it is most common among those over the age of 65, hence the name 'age-related.' Age-related macular degeneration afflicts both eyes fairly equally, but can develop in one eye earlier than the other.

The Macula

First, here is a brief explanation as to what the macula is and why it is so important:

The macula is found in the back of the eye, as a part of the retina. It is a very small area where specialized nerve cells, called cones, are compacted tightly together. These cones are connected to the brain through the optic nerve. The brain has selected the macula as the area to point in the direction to view, because of its structure and sensitivity to detecting line and form. This is our 'high-definition' area that gives us our best vision (referred to as best visual acuity.)

The macula is a very small, very sensitive, and a very specialized area of the retina. It also has the highest rate of metabolism, and therefore is highly sensitive to blood flow and nutritional supply. Therein lies the source of the vision problems. Aging and poor health (such as high blood pressure and vascular disease), when combined with environmental factors (such as smoking and excessive UV exposure), and perhaps hereditary factors, can lead to degeneration of this very sensitive area, resulting in macular degeneration.

Signs and Symptoms

Age-related macular degeneration is divided into two major categories: 1. wet ARMD and 2. dry ARMD.

Dry ARMD

The onset of dry ARMD is a slow, insidious change in vision, such as blurring and/or distortion (lines are not straight). The initial changes may not even be noticed when viewing with both eyes, as one eye may compensate for the other. The first sign may be seen by your eye care professional. The doctor may see only a subtle color change or small yellow deposits called drusen, in the macular area. Drusen are the waste products of the macula's metabolism. They indicate changes in the macula, and that the macula can no longer remove or recycle these waste products efficiently. They have now begun to accumulate. This accumulation of byproducts of metabolism is toxic to the cells, which protect the vital cones of the macula. After the toxic accumulation of drusen comes the death of these cells. The death of cells means a decrease in the capability of the macula to detect fine lines and forms. The result is a loss of visual acuity. The process can be slow, taking years before serious debilitating vision loss occurs.

The causes of dry macular degeneration are still a matter of clinical research. It is believed there is no one mechanism, but possibly a combination of heredity, general health, and environmental factors.

Treatment

The loss of vision is not reversible. What is recommended for dry macular degeneration is a means for slowing the progression of vision loss. In the early stages, lifestyle changes, such as quitting smoking, better diet, and exercise are recommended. Sunglasses should be worn to decrease the amount of potentially damaging UV light to the very sensitive macula.

You can also purchase nutriceuticals to provide needed nutrients as supplements to a diet that might not provide enough of the essential vitamins for eye health.

Wet ARMD

The wet form differs from dry ARMD by a more rapid onset

and an equally rapid loss of vision, if untreated. It is less common than the dry form. About 10 percent of people with dry macular degeneration will convert to wet ARMD. Unlike dry ARMD, there is an accumulation of blood or fluid beneath the macula, rather than the slow accumulation of waste products This disease is most commonly found in those with vascular disease.

In the early stage of wet ARMD there is a loss of visual acuity, distortion, and possibly, color perception changes. A complicating factor is the growth of abnormal blood vessels underneath the macula. This growth of new, abnormal blood vessels is called neovascularization. These blood vessels grow in response to low oxygen levels in the retina. The fragile blood vessels are susceptible to breakage and leakage, which results in more fluid and blood in the macula. These pockets of fluid and/or blood are damaging and toxic to the vital cells that support the macula.

Treatment

The treatment for the wet form of ARMD requires timely detection and intervention by the eye doctor. Treatment during the early stages, although it will not reverse damage already done to the central vision area, can reduce the severity of vision loss. There are three techniques to halt the growth of abnormal blood vessels, thereby limiting potential damage:

1. Injection Only. Injection into the eye of a drug that stops the development of new, weak and fragile blood vessels. The drug is called anti-VEGF. VEGF (vascular endothelial growth factor) is produced by the oxygen starved tissues of the eye to promote

the abnormal blood vessel growth. Although growing new blood vessels seems like a good idea, these new blood vessels are problematic in that they are fragile. The anti-VEGF drug injection stops the growth to alleviate the problem.

2. Injection and Laser. The drug is injected into the arm and within minutes is taken up by the fragile new vessels of the macula. The injection is followed by a laser treatment to the affected area of the eye to activate the drug. The drug then closes off the abnormal blood vessels to stop the growth and subsequent leaking and bleeding. This is called photodynamic therapy. This treatment is not permanent, and may need to be repeated in three months.

3. Laser Only. Laser treatment is done around the area of the macula that in effect destroys the surrounding leaky blood vessels. It is not likely to be done in the macular area, as it can destroy the sensitive retinal cells above the targeted blood vessels, leaving a little blind spot. This is called photocoagulation laser therapy.

All three of these treatments are done in the retina specialist's office on an outpatient basis.

Self Monitoring

A proactive approach for those who have been identified as being at risk for macular degeneration is to self-monitor at home, on a daily basis. The Amsler grid (a copy can be found in the appendix) is the standard form given to patients for this purpose. When observing the grid, any changes that deviates from the straightness of the lines or the regularity of the squares, is an indicator of macular disruption and change in vision. In this way, a person can identify early changes they may not otherwise notice. Be proactive, be your own advocate!

Low Vision Strategies

The resulting vision for both wet and dry forms of macular degeneration is loss of the central 4 to 10 degrees of vision. Most affected are those activities that involve detailed vision, like reading, writing, driving, and facial recognition. Macular degeneration does not result in total blindness. As devastating as the loss of central vision is, people with vision loss secondary to ARMD still have a lot of retina that is still viable and useful. This peripheral retina, although not as sensitive as the macula for detail, is sensitive to light and motion. Because of that, those with ARMD are able to use assistive technology.

Management

Those with MD benefit from:

1. Good Illumination. Work areas should have adequate task lighting that is directed at the surface. An over the shoulder lamp directed at reading material is helpful.

2. Sunglasses. These help increase contrast, glare reduction, and protect the eyes from the damaging effects of UV light.

3. Hats with brims. Hats help with glare reduction.

4. Magnification. Bigger is better. This is a very broad category.

Start first with an optimal set of near eyeglasses, determined for you by a patient eye care professional. They can help determine a prescription that enables you to bring printed material closer. When things are closer, they appear bigger.

Next, adapt your environment to your needs. Look for larger printed books, magazines, phones, TV remotes, TV screens, computer keyboards, etc. Finally, in the bigger is better category, those with MD do well with magnifying devices.

5. Telescopes and Bioptics. Distance objects can be made to appear larger and closer through the use of lens systems. The telescope can either be hand-held, or mounted into eyeglasses. A bioptic is a small telescope mounted in a high position in the prescription lens. These are commonly prescribed for those who still qualify for driving privileges.

6. Rehabilitative Services. Remember macular degeneration leaves the rest of the retina intact. If unable to learn on your own, rehabilitative training can teach eccentric fixation. When using eccentric fixation, essentially the 'blind' macula is moved out of the way and another part of the retina is used for viewing. This is done by shifting the central area slightly up, down, or to the left. (Shifting to the right makes reading more difficult.) It is a technique that takes practice. (For more information see the chapter on Adaptive Techniques). An individual who loses their vision over a long period of time may find this technique on their own. You will also need magnification, as these areas

are less sensitive than the macula.

7. Nutritional Supplements. The National Eye Institute and the National Institute for Health conducted a study that looked at the benefit of taking supplements for eye disease, called the Age-Related Eye Disease Study (AREDS). They evaluated various combinations of antioxidants, lutein, zeaxanthin, and zinc. They concluded that the "AREDS 2 combination of supplements had the benefit of slowing the progression for advanced stages of macular degeneration."

   The AREDS 2 formula included:
   - 500 milligrams (mg) of vitamin C
   - 400 international units (IU) of vitamin E
   - 25 mg zinc as zinc oxide
   - 10 mg lutein and 2 mg zeaxanthin
   - 1000 mg omega-3 fatty acids
     (350mg DHA and 650mg EPA)
   - 2 mg of copper as copper oxide

This particular combination can be purchased as commercially available 'eye vitamins' or as 'AREDS formula.' Consult your medical doctor and eye care professional before launching into a long-term supplement program to determine if it is right for you. (Complications associated with taking zinc have been reported.)

Additional Reading:

- National Eye Institute Age-Related Macular Degeneration. **www.nei.nih.gov/health/maculardegen/armd_facts.as**

Home>>Health Information>> Facts about Age-Related Macular Degeneration.

- Macular Degeneration Research and Information. Brighthouse Foundation. **www.brightfocus.org/macular/**.
- Age-Related Macular Degeneration. VisionAware **www.visionaware.org**.
- MD Support. **www.mdsupport.org/**
- Age-Related Eye Disease Study 2. (AREDS2) **www.nei.nih.gov/areds2/**. For the Public: What the Age-Related Eye Disease Studies Mean for You.

Cataracts

When a senior patient came into my office complaining of vision problems, the most common diagnosis was cataracts, especially if they keep taking their glasses off and repeatedly cleaning them because they are 'dirty.' The good news is that cataracts is one of the treatable forms of vision loss.

The lens of the eye is where cataracts form. The lens is found where you would expect to find the lens in a camera. It is located behind a diaphragm that opens and closes. In the eye, the iris is the diaphragm.

The lens of the eye at birth starts out crystal clear and has the capability to flex, which is how the eye is able to focus from distance to near. (There are, however, hereditary forms of cataracts.) Soon thereafter, the lens begins to age. By the time we are in our 40s, it hardens down to the point where we can no longer flex the lens to focus. This is a sign of lens aging and is the point at which we must resign ourselves to getting our first set of reading eyeglasses.

As the lens of the eye continues to age, it becomes harder and denser, taking on color or cloudiness. Anything that is less than clear is considered a cataract. Having said that, however, not all cataracts are significant, and not all cataracts are detrimental to vision. There is not just one type of cataract; there are actually numerous types. Some have a rapid onset; whereas others take years to develop to the point where they impact a person's day to day functioning.

Risk Factors

The most common risk factor for the development of cataracts is age. Health issues such as poor nutrition, diabetes, smoking, and alcohol abuse can promote cataract formation. Some medications, such as corticosteroids have been implicated as a cause of cataract formation. Environmental factors, such as UV light exposure, have also been studied as sources of cataract genesis. UV damage can stem from intense sunlight exposure, as in latitude (closer to the equator) or chronic sunlight exposure (occupational, like fishing). Trauma to the eye can cause rapid cataract formation, or the cataract can occur years later as a reminder of the incident.

Types of Cataracts

These different factors cause different types of lens opacities. The type of cataract determines how visual acuity is affected. There are three general types.

1. Nuclear Sclerotic Cataract

This is the most common type of cataract. As the lens gets harder and denser, it takes on an amber color. At this point, the vision may still be 20/20, but the eyeglass prescription may change. (Your doctor may even say to you that your eyeglass prescription is 'better.') You might find yourself holding reading material closer, and that more light is required to see better. Interestingly, your vision outdoors is great; it is indoors that is the problem. But as time passes (maybe years) the amber color of the lens becomes darker, and takes on a brownish hue (brunescence). The doctor can no longer change your prescription to give you 20/20 vision, and the world has now taken on a dim hazy appearance.

2. Cortical Cataracts

'Cortical' indicates cataracts within the cortex of the lens. They can be anterior cortical, posterior cortical, or both. The appearance can vary from 'crack–like' lines, vacuoles (like bubbles), or generalized haze. Because of these lens imperfections, light entering the eye will be scattered, and there is a perception of glare. They are most evident at night as star patterns around lights. Vision is decreased because there is no clear pathway for light to enter the eye. Stepping into sunlight makes it all the worse.

This type of cataract tends to be slow growing. Often cortical cataracts will start on the edges of the lens and grow toward the center. Your eye doctor may be able to visualize them, in the early stages, only when the pupil is dilated to expose the edges of the lens.

3. Posterior Sub-Capsular Cataracts

The lens of the eye rests in a membrane capsule that holds the lens in place. It is here, at the backside of the lens, just in front of this capsule, where the fastest growing cataract occurs. It appears to your doctor as a hazy grainy area on the backside of the lens. In as quickly as several months, it can have a devastating effect on vision.

Side View of a Lens:

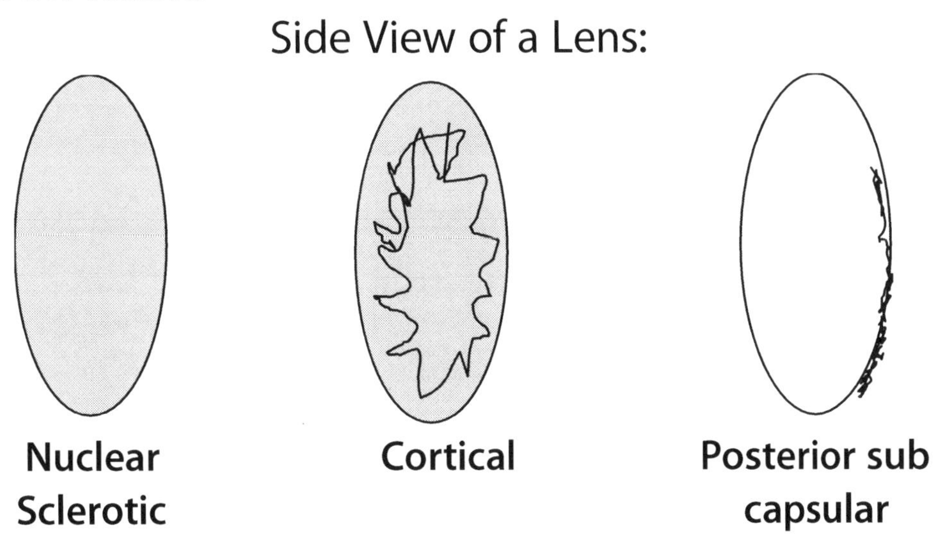

Signs and Symptoms

There is a lot of variability as to how cataracts will affect vision, and in the rate of growth. Cataracts affect both eyes, but may affect one eye sooner than the other. Generally, glare or halos around lights and/or a decrease in visual acuity are the first signs. The glare from daylight or oncoming headlights of cars can cause discomfort. The haziness of the lens makes the environment look washed out or low in contrast. The feeling is that your eyeglasses are dirty or that you are looking through a dirty windshield. Often these changes are very slow and insidious, and may not be noticed until it affects your ability to function.

Treatment

The good news is that cataracts are treatable and cataract surgery has evolved to outpatient one-day surgery status. Provided there is no other eye disease, good visual acuity can be achieved. Surgeons will determine, with the help of pre-op testing, the best lens implants for the patient. With the proper implant, distance prescriptions can be reduced down to a minimum, with good visual recovery. Only reading glasses may be required. Even on that issue, there are options for multifocal intra-ocular lens implants that reduce the need for glasses to read. However, these premium lenses may not be covered by insurance.

Management

If surgery is not an option, there are a few things the patient and doctor can do to help with day to day activities:

1. Stronger eyeglasses that give some magnification;
2. Illuminated hand held and stand magnifiers or illuminated electronic magnifiers for viewing small details;
3. Sunglasses and brimmed hats to reduce glare; and
4. Adequate interior lighting.

Additional Reading:

- Facts About Cataracts. National Eye Institute. **www.nei.nih.gov/**.
- Cataracts. American Optometric Association Glossary of all Eye and Vision conditions. **www.aoa.org/**.
- Cataracts. VisionAware. **www.visionaware.org**.

Diabetic Eye Disease

Diabetes is a group of chronic diseases that affect how blood sugar (specifically glucose), is metabolized, or not metabolized, by the body. This inability to utilize blood sugar results in high levels of glucose in the blood vessels, which ultimately damages the integrity of the blood vessels. Those individuals that suffer from diabetes should be educated by their medical professionals that controlling and monitoring blood sugar level is important for guarding the well being of the kidneys, the eyes, and the peripheral blood vessels, especially of the feet. These three areas are of most concern because their functioning is dependent on the health of very small blood vessels which are susceptible to damage from poorly controlled blood sugar. Regular visits to the medical doctor, podiatrist, and eye doctor become a way of life.

The great benefit of regular eye exams is that the eye is the only place in the body that a doctor can actually see the blood vessels. Ocular blood vessels are small and are called 'terminal blood vessels.' If the blood vessels of a diabetic begin to leak, the eye is the first place where the damage can be seen, even before the diabetic notices any change in vision. The damaging changes of leaking, bleeding, abnormal blood vessel growth (neovascularization), macular swelling (macular edema), and finally, scarring, are all a part of what is called diabetic retinopathy. Diabetics are also at risk for developing cataracts and glaucoma.

Signs and Symptoms

Eye doctors use a grading system for the stages of diabetic retinopathy as a guideline for treatment and management of their diabetic patients.

- Non-Proliferative Diabetic Retinopathy (NPDR). Often in the early stages, there is no change in vision. A patient may be unaware that blood sugar is extracting a toll on the integrity of their retinal blood vessels. Sometimes the first sign will be blurred or fluctuating vision. Next, there may be some loss of visual acuity. It is through a dilated eye examination that these early signs of diabetic changes can be seen. The doctor will note small hemorrhages, also called micro-hemorrhages, and macular swelling, also known as macular edema. The swelling of the macula may be accompanied by distortion of vision. This early stage of diabetic retinopathy is called non-proliferative diabetic retinopathy (NPDR).
- Proliferative Diabetic Retinopathy (PDR). This next stage is more severe and detrimental to vision. PDR is identified as a 'proliferation' of blood vessels. Not only may there be blurring and fluctuations in vision, but there may also be

more floaters and blind spots. What the doctor looks for during a dilated eye examination is abnormal vessel growth (neovascularization), larger hemorrhages, areas of vessel leakage, and macular swelling. The retina has become starved for oxygen flow, due to the damage to the blood vessels feeding it. This whole cascade of uncontrolled blood sugar results in blood vessel damage with leaking and bleeding, then new vessel growth, then the subsequent death of the photoreceptor cells (light sensitive cells), and vision loss.

Diabetes can affect other aspects of vision, beyond the retinal damage. It may cause problems with dark adaption and color vision. Diabetics can suffer with dry eye syndrome, which has symptoms of irritated, red, scratchy, and a gritty feeling. Cataracts of the lens may form from taking on fluid and swelling. Glaucoma may develop due to abnormal blood vessel growth which blocks the outflow of fluid from the eye.

Diabetic eye disease progression varies from person to person in that it can range from no visual changes, to progressing from mild vision loss, to moderate vision loss, to severe vision loss, and the possibility of blindness.

Treatment

"An ounce of prevention is worth a pound of cure." Careful monitoring and management of blood sugar levels by the patient, accompanied by frequent (every six months) comprehensive eye examinations, to watch for early signs of diabetic retinopathy, have been proven to slow the progression of diabetic retinopathy and prevent vision loss. (Early Treatment of Diabetic Retinopathy Study (ETDRS).). High blood pressure, which is a risk factor for diabetic retinopathy, should be controlled. Diabetics also benefit from weight control, cessation of smoking, and lifestyle changes.

Treatment depends on the severity, and it is not a cure. Treatment is about preservation of the retina and prevention of blindness. If proliferative diabetic retinopathy develops; laser treatment is warranted to stem the bleeding and oxygen demand of the retina to prevent the development of neovascularization and preservation of the central macular area. Retina specialists can inject an anti-vascular endothelial growth factor (anti-VEGF) into the eyes of those with macular edema, to prevent the growth of the abnormal fragile blood vessels that can destroy the central vision.

A vitrectomy may be preformed to remove the gelatin- like fluid in the eye. This is done if there has been blood vessel growth and/or a significant bleed into the central cavity of the eye. The removal of the vitreous is done to prevent scar tissue formation, which can result in retinal detachment. These treatments have been successful in helping diabetic patients maintain vision.

Keep in mind, the longer a person has diabetes, the greater the chance for developing changes associated with diabetic eye disease. Diligent control of this chronic disease is a lifelong process.

Management

People who have lost vision to diabetic retinopathy benefit from:

1. Magnifiers. It is best to select those magnifying aids that can

be adjusted should there be a progression of vision loss.

2. Sunglasses. These are used to increase contrast, glare reduction, and protect the eyes from the damaging effects of UV light.

3. Good Interior Lighting. Work areas should have adequate task lighting that is directed at the surface. An over the shoulder lamp directed at reading material is helpful.

4. Modified Diabetic Care Aids. There are magnifiers for syringes to magnify the syringe markings. Glucometers can be found that have large digital readout, or are 'talking' glucometers, which give audio readings. Large print diabetic log books can also be helpful.

5. Rehabilitative Services. Therapists can help with making changes to the home environment to help with adaption.

6. Orientation and Mobility Training. This service is helpful for the severely impaired.

Additional Reading:

- American Diabetes Association. **www.diabetes.org/**
- Facts About Diabetic Eye Disease. NEI Health Information. **www.nei.nih.gov/health/diabetic/retinopathy.asp**.
- Diabetic Retinopathy. VisionAware. **www.visionaware.org**.

Glaucoma

Glaucoma is a thief. It is a disease process that silently steals vision, and, with the exception of the acute form, there is no pain or visual disturbances. You don't even know you have it, unless an eye doctor identifies the disease. Glaucoma is another reason to get regular eye examinations.

Glaucoma is a general term, used to describe numerous subgroups of the eye disease that result in optic nerve damage. The simple definition is that it is a disease of high eye pressure, but it is actually more complicated than that. Occasionally, a patient may come in to the doctor's office with very high eye pressure, and the diagnosis of glaucoma is a slam dunk. More commonly, it can be difficult to diagnose. The doctor must look at and evaluate many factors. Eye pressure tests are performed, photographs may be taken, visual field tests are completed, and Ocular Coherence Tomography (OCT), are all done and evaluated.

In the early stages, the doctor may request all these tests be repeated in three to six months. The results are then reviewed and compared. This process of repeat testing may go on for months or years. The doctor is looking for a progression, and if found, treatment can begin before there is significant vision loss.

The problem of glaucoma is related to outflow of aqueous fluid from the eye. The eye is constantly manufacturing fluid in the anterior chamber of the eye. This fluid continually flows out of the eye by way of the blood stream. The disease of glaucoma occurs as a result of a disruption in the flow of the fluid out of the eye. The type of glaucoma is based on the underlying cause of the disease.

The damage of glaucoma is evident at the optic nerve, which is where the light sensitive nerves of the retina come together and exit the orbit of the eye on their way to the brain. It is the changes to the optic nerve that the doctor evaluates to diagnose, and then manage the treatment. It is a disease that cannot be prevented or cured (except for the acute form). It is chronic, progressive, lifelong, and potentially blinding if not treated.

Glaucoma has several subcategories. Chief among them are: primary open angle glaucoma, acute angle closure, the secondary glaucomas, and congenital glaucoma. The subtypes of glaucoma:

1. Primary Open Angle Glaucoma (POAG). This is the most common form of glaucoma. The causes are not completely understood, and are still a matter of research. Sometimes it is related to high pressure within the eye, and sometimes it is not. What is known, are the risk factors. Those over the age of 60 are at risk for developing glaucoma. African Americans have a higher risk and can develop it at a younger age. Family history, means that close blood relatives, who have been diagnosed with glaucoma, are an indication that other family members need to be monitored for the early detection of glaucoma.

2. The Secondary Glaucomas. Glaucoma can be caused by other factors that affect the eye. Factors include systemic disease, medications, trauma, and inflammation. There are two other anomalies called Pigmentary Dispersion and Pseudoexfoliative Syndrome that can progress to cause glaucoma by a mechanical blockage of fluid outflow.

3. Acute Angle Closure Glaucoma. This is the most symptomatic form and the most treatable form of glaucoma. Acute angle

closure is an ocular emergency, with symptoms such as pain, headache, nausea, blurred vision, and halos around lights. In primary open angle glaucoma, eye pressure goes up because of resistance to the outflow of aqueous fluid from the eye in a slow progressive manner. Angle closure glaucoma is the result of a mechanical closure of the outflow area by the iris with a rapid rise in eye pressure. Angle closure can be cured by a laser treatment that opens a drainage hole in the iris, called an iridotomy. The sooner treatment is initiated, the better the visual outcome.

4. Congenital Glaucoma. This form of glaucoma is present at birth, but may not be diagnosed until months or even years later. The signs are of an infant with large appearing eyes, hazy cornea, tearing, and light sensitivity. The cause may be primary, meaning that the area where fluid outflows from the eye, is not formed properly. Secondary forms of congenital glaucoma may be associated with other inherited diseases, such as malformations of the eye, or part of a larger systemic syndrome like Prader-Willi Syndrome, fetal alcohol syndrome, or Rubella. Unlike adult onset glaucoma, surgery is the first line of treatment in most cases.

Signs and Symptoms

In the early stages of POAG and the secondary glaucomas there are no signs or symptoms. It is not until the moderate or severe stages of the disease sets in that there may be detectable vision loss. The first sign might be that objects seem to jump in or out of view, or parts of objects may be missing. The appearance and disappearance of objects is because of visual field loss and/or blind spots in the retina due to nerve cell death. An example is an inability to see another car to the side when driving, or bumping into door jams because there is some loss of peripheral vision. A whole sector of vision may be lost, in one eye, but not initially noticed because the visual field of the other eye compensates. Glaucoma generally affects both eyes, but is often initially diagnosed in one eye.

Glaucoma attacks from the mid-peripheral vision areas of the eye, working its way to the central macular area. Throughout the course of the disease, 20/20 vision can be maintained. The macula may be spared until the very end.

Treatment

The treatment of glaucoma is not only science but is an art. The management and treatment goal of treating glaucoma is to slow the progression and stabilize the visual field loss.

Medical treatment has several stages:

1. Eye Drops. Eye drops function in one of two ways:
    - Decrease the production of aqueous fluid, (ex: beta-blockers); or
    - Increase outflow of fluid, (ex: prostaglandins).

   The eye drops may be prescribed singly or several to be used in combination. The pressure of the eye and the welfare of the optic nerve are closely monitored to gauge the effectiveness of the eye drop treatment to preserve peripheral vision. Other types of drops may be added or withdrawn. That is the art of glaucoma management.

2. Laser Treatment. When, over a period of time, the doctor decides that the eye drops are not effective enough in halting the damage, laser treatment is the next step. The laser is directed at the angle where the iris meets the cornea and conjunctiva. Here is where the trabeculum drains the fluid of the eye. The laser treatment 'opens up the drain,' by poking holes in the trabeculum. The idea is if the drainage is open, it will increase fluid outflow to decrease the pressure. This treatment may have to be done several times, as the benefit may last about 3 years.

3. Surgical Intervention and the Filtering Drain. There are several techniques to increase the outflow of fluid. One microsurgical technique opens a passage to the conjunctival area. There, a bleb (bubble-like), is formed on the surface of the conjunctiva, where fluid from the eye escapes. Another surgical technique opens up the passage to form a direct connection to the outflow canal within the eye.

Compliance and the Glaucoma Patient

In the early stages of glaucoma, the go- to-treatment is the use of eye drops to control eye pressure. Patients and doctors struggle with the issue of compliance. If glaucoma is diagnosed early and a patient has no significant vision loss and no symptoms, there may be little motivation on the part of the patient to keep up with the eye drop regimen. Eye drops are instilled once every day, sometimes twice a day. The more moderate and severe cases may require several drops at different times of day, and perhaps the addition of an oral medication. The patient may perceive this as inconvenient. There can be side effects such as burning and stinging. Some people, no matter how hard they try, cannot seem to get those eye drops into the eye. There may be financial concerns, as the medications can be expensive. These factors can add up to a patient either being lackadaisical or resistant to keeping up the daily regimen. The doctor has to deal with patients (here I will apologize in advance) that…lie. (Sorry, it needs to be said.) Patients claim compliance, but often fall short. Staying on course with glaucoma treatment can be tough. The importance of regular instillation of medications cannot be emphasized enough. It will determine the success of the therapy.

Management: Low Vision and Glaucoma

How glaucoma affects vision varies from person to person. Someone in the early stages of glaucoma, who has some visual field loss that does not affect how they function with activities of daily living, will not perceive a need for low vision aids. However, a person who has more severe visual field loss will benefit from:

1. Scanning. Techniques can be learned to efficiently and effectively scan an environment to get the whole picture.
2. Specialty Aids for Field Enhancement. Although nothing can completely replace the loss of visual field, lens add-ons such

as Fresnel prisms and mirrors can be placed on the glasses, in the area of field loss, to give an enhanced access to viewing objects in the area of vision loss.

3. Field Expanders. This takes the form of reversing a low power telescope, or viewing through a concave lens. Both minimize the environment, thereby expanding the area seen. Unfortunately, it does make details smaller and more difficult to see.

   Both field enhancers and field expanders need to be prescribed and fitted by a low vision professional. Remember, nothing can take the place of lost visual field. These aids are used intermittently and briefly to access the environment. There will be some training and adaption required.

4. Reading and Writing Guides. Those who have problems following print, because of visual field loss, can benefit from using a guide. This is a dark plastic or cardboard plate, with an open slotted area, that the user slides along the line of print they are trying to read. Our peripheral vision normally helps guide us when reading. The guide helps those with a constricted visual field to find their way across the page.

5. Rehabilitative Services. Therapists can help with making changes to the home environment to help with adaption.

6. Orientation and Mobility Training. Those with the most severe, constricting visual field loss will benefit from training with an Orientation and Mobility Specialist to better negotiate their environment.

Additional Reading:

- Facts About Glaucoma NEI Health Information **https://www.nei.nih.gov/**.
- Glaucoma Research Foundation. **www.glaucoma.org/**.
- Glaucoma Research and Information. BrightFocus Foundation. **www.brightfocus.org/glaucoma/.**

Optic Neuropathy

Optic neuropathy is a general term used to describe vision loss due to optic nerve damage. The causes are a broad category of diseases that affect the optic nerve anywhere from the optic nerve head inside the eyeball, back to the visual cortex of the brain. The amount of vision loss is variable depending on the underlying cause.

The categories are:

Rapid Onset:

1. Inflammatory Diseases. These include: sarcoid, systemic lupus, and inflammatory bowel disease.
2. Demyelinating Diseases. For example: multiple sclerosis,
3. Vascular Diseases. These include: Giant cell arthritis and diabetes.
4. Infectious Diseases. This includes: Lyme disease, Cat Scratch Disease.
5. Traumatic. Vision loss is caused by: blunt head or eye trauma.

Slower, Progressive Onset:

1. Obstructive/Compressive. These include: growths within the eye orbit or brain such as: gliomas, adenoma of the pituitary gland, and meningiomas.

2. Toxic/Nutritional. This includes: Methanol and ethanol toxicity, or vitamin deficiencies.

3. Hereditary. This includes: Leber's Mitochondrial Optic Neuropathy and inherited optic atrophy.

The light sensitive neurons (photoreceptors) have fibrils that traverse the retina and come together at the optic nerve. These fibrils are bundled together in a cable-like fashion and extend out of the eyeball as the optic nerve, all the way to the back of the brain, where the visual cortex lies. Optic neuropathy results from a disturbance somewhere along this pathway.

A disease causing optic neuropathy may affect only one eye, but depending on the underlying cause, can progress to affect both eyes. The degree to which vision is affected is dependent on the cause, duration, and in some cases the expediency of treatment.

Signs and symptoms

The vision loss may be of sudden onset or a slower progressive change in vision. What the doctor nay see upon initial examination is a swollen optic nerve (optic neuritis), pale optic nerve (optic atrophy), or nothing. The diagnosis will be made based on history, other associated signs and symptoms, and a battery of tests to find the cause.

Initially, the visual disturbance may be a total or partial loss of vision, accompanied by blur, flashes, distortion of vision, changes in color perception, and/or generalized dimming and loss of contrast sensitivity. There may or may not be any pain depending on the cause.

There can be blind spots called scotomas. These scotomas can be a large sector visual field loss, or small areas. Where the scotoma is will determine the degree of vision loss. Neuropathy that includes the central macula area will have the most devastating effect on the visual outcome.

Color perception changes are most evident in the reds. The color red may have a pale or washed out appearance.

The loss of vision may be followed by a resolution of the disease process and some visual recovery over a period of weeks or months. Any permanent vision loss is a result of the damage that remains.

Treatment

Because optic neuropathy is a broad category of disease processes, the treatment will depend on a careful diagnosis by your specialist. Treatment will involve a team approach which includes the eye care professional and a medical professional specializing in the underlying disease process.

Management

What your low vision specialist can do, in the event of bilateral vision loss:

1. Magnifiers. Those who have lost central vision will benefit by the use of magnifying aids.

2. Tints and Filters on Lenses. This will help with color vision and contrast.

3. Good Illumination. This will help with work and tasks of daily living.

4. Vision Rehabilitation Training. This can help to develop adaptive strategies for visual field loss.

5. Orientation and Mobility Training. This is for the more severely impaired to help them better negotiate their environment.

Bibliography

1. Alexander, Larry J. OD: Primary Care of the Posterior Segment. West Norwalk, Connecticut/San Mateo, California. Appleton & Lange, 1989.

2. Behbehani, Raed. Clinical Approach to Optic Neuropathies. Clinical Ophthalmology. Auckland, NZ. 2007, September, 1(3): 233-246.

3. Lewis, Thomas L., Fingeret, Murray. Primary Care of the Glaucomas. Norwalk, Connecticut. Appleton & Lange, 1993.

4. Marks, Esther S., Adamczyk, Diane T., Thomann, Kelly H. Primary Eye care in Systemic Disease. Norwalk, Connecticut. Appleton & Lange, 1995.

5. Nowakowski, Rodney W.; Primary Low Vision Care, Norwalk, Connecticut. Appleton& Lange, 1994.

6. Pelino, Carlo J., OD, Pizzimenti, Joseph J., OD. Contemporary Care Protocols for DR and DME. Review of Optometry. 2012, August 15, Vol. 149, No. 8, 90-97.

Inherited Eye Diseases

Inherited means the passing of genetic information by way of parent to offspring. Each parent contributes half of the genetic material needed for a life form to take shape.

The egg from the mother, and the sperm of the father each have 22 chromosomes and one sex chromosome. The chromosomes form the long strands that carry genetic information which is called DNA. The union of egg and sperm completes the pairing of the chromosomes. Now the central cell 'factory,' called the nucleus, has the needed 46 total chromosomes aligned as 22 pairs and a set of sex chromosomes (XX for female, XY for males).

The 22 pairs of chromosomes are called autosomes. The genetic code is the complex DNA pattern of thousands of genes. Alterations in normal, functional gene coding are termed mutations. It is these mutations that give rise to errors that we call disease.

The classification of hereditary diseases is not simple. Some are a single gene disease called monogenic (like Stargardt's disease) or complex (like glaucoma and age-related macular degeneration), which can involve different genes or multiples of genes. The disease can be limited to just the eye (Retinitis pigmentosa) or as a syndrome (Ushers disease in which retinitis pigmentosa is a component). A hereditary eye disease can affect a young person in their first or second decade of life, or it can lay in wait to set in at a later age, as a progressive disease.

The terms frequently referred to in the discussion of hereditary diseases are the terms autosomal dominant, autosomal recessive, and X-linked. Keep in mind for the following discussion that the autosome is a pair of chromosomes, one from each parent, and each chromosome comes with its own set of genes (codes for different characteristics).

Inheritance Patterns

Autosomal Dominant

The characteristics associated with a disease termed autosomal dominant are:

1. Single gene diseases in which only one of two genes are needed for the disorder to be manifest.
2. Usually one parent is affected by the disorder.
3. The disorder may manifest in every generation.
4. Chance of inheriting the disorder is generally 50 percent.

Autosomal Recessive

The characteristics associated with a disease termed autosomal recessive are:

1. Two genes are needed for the disorder to manifest.
2. Parents may be unaffected by the disorder.

3. Parents are both 'carriers,' meaning they both have a single gene for the disorder, but because it is recessive, they are not affected.

4. The offspring have a 25 percent chance of inheriting the disorder.

   Keep in mind, the percentages indicate that each child born has a 50 percent or 25 percent chance of developing the disease, **not** necessarily 50 percent or 25 percent of the children born will have the disorder.

X-Linked (Sex-Chromosome Linked)

The inheritance pattern for the sex chromosome is an X chromosome from the mother, and either an X or a Y chromosome from the father. Females have two X chromosomes (XX) and males have one X and one Y chromosome (XY). Therefore, the father's contribution determines the sex of the child.

The general characteristics of an x-linked chromosome disorder are:

1. Generally, the mutations are on the X chromosome.

2. Disorders can affect males and females in each generation.

3. Patterns of X-linked chromosome disorders have more complicated inheritance patterns. Who will develop the disorder depends on the sex of the affected parent, sex of the 'carrier' parent, and the sex of the offspring.

Additional Reading

- The website of the National Human Genome Research

Institute has an excellent 'Talking Glossary of Terms.' National Human Genome Research Institute >> Education >>Talking Glossary of Terms. **www.genome.gov/Education/**.

- A detailed description of inheritance patterns can be found at the website of the National Library of Medicine, National Institute of Health Medline Plus Encyclopedia, Medline Plus >>Medical Encyclopedia. **www.nlm.nih.gov/medlineplus/encyclopedia.html**.

Human Genome Project

Genetic testing is slowly becoming a part of contemporary medicine due to the extensive research and discovery of the Human Genome Project.

The Human Genome Project was a US government funded study, whose goal was to map the sequence of molecular basis of the human DNA (human genetic code). The project officially began in 1990 and was completed in 2003. The project not only mapped the human genome, but was able to determine gene functions for the production of different proteins. It is how these genes function that determines an individual's physical features and biological function.

Thanks to the National Center for Human Genome Research Institute, an international consortium of researchers, and the commitment of the US government to share its discoveries, the technology and database of the Human Genome Project is made available to the public. Gene testing for hundreds of inherited eye diseases is now possible.

The project also developed improved technology for gene research and testing. The results of the Human Genome Project are far reaching, and have already influenced medicine in terms of early detection, diagnosis, treatment, and research to find cures. It is projected that with continued research and discovery, medicine will one day be customized to the individual based on genetics.

Additional Reading

- To learn more about the Human Genome Project: National Human Genome Research Institute >> Education>>About the Human Genome Project at **http://www.genome.gov/10001772**

Genetic Testing

The specimen used for the genetic analysis is usually blood, saliva, or a buccal swab (swab from the inside cheek of the mouth). The laboratory test looks at the molecular level to analyze an individual's genetic makeup; to confirm if there is a variation in the DNA sequence. That variation can be in the form of an addition, a deletion, a substitution, or duplication. Then based on probability, gleaned from the database of other persons with the same genetic variation, it is determined if this variation is a mutation that is disease causing. It is a probability, because not all variations result in disease.(1)

The easiest genetic variations to determine are those that are monogenic. These variations result in diseases that are due to changes in just one gene.

Complex genetic diseases require analyses of multiple DNA segments. What the variation is, and how these genes interact, determine the disease process. These complex genetic diseases can be more difficult to decipher.

There are several reasons to perform genetic testing. Deciding to undergo genetic testing is best determined by its 'meaningfulness.'(1,2) It is meaningful if a definitive diagnosis is needed to determine management and treatment options, should there be any. In the early stages of a disease. It is meaningful to be able to 'rule in' or 'rule out' a disease, and knowing can help with understanding the disease prognosis and to be able to anticipate the future. Parents, who have a family history of a particular disease, may want to know if they are carriers of the gene for that disease, as it may influence their decisions for having children. Those individuals, who anticipate being part of a research project, although they have a clinical diagnosis, may need to undergo genetic testing for the study. These are all meaningful reasons to have genetic testing done.

A disease that has already been diagnosed by way of clinical findings, and treatment options has already been determined based on these findings, in this case, genetic testing is not going to change anything. Therefore, the genetic test results lack meaningfulness.

When considering genetic testing, consider not only the medical benefits listed above, but consider the psychological impact. There may be a sense of relief, having a definitive diagnosis, with its associated prognosis. The feeling may be one of purposefulness, in that now you understand and can move forward. (Knowledge is power.) The flip side is the fear, stress, and anxiety that comes with knowing it is an inherited progressive disease. There can be the feeling of guilt and changes in family relationships.(3)

There are direct-to-consumer genetic testing kits available. These are tests that you can order without going through a medical professional. These can be found on the internet. The benefits of these involves privacy, and that they are less expensive. Most direct-to-consumer tests are for ancestral lineage or general-health related genetics. You will be hard pressed to find direct-to-consumer genetic testing for the rarer eye diseases. The issue with this route is that you need to know what you are ordering, and how to interpret the results. Consider also, the psychosocial aspects, and the meaningfulness for diagnosis and prognosis. For those reasons, it is best to combine genetic testing with the expertise of a medical geneticist and/or genetic counselor. (4)

Additional Resources

- Genetic testing by way of a registered medical professional: eyeGENE , a division of the National Eye Institute. **https://www.nei.nih.gov/eyegene/**.
- For more information before ordering your own direct-to-consumer genetic test, see: Direct to Consumer Genetic Tests, Consumer Information at the Federal Trade Commission Website: **www.consumer.ftc.gov/**.

Genetic Counseling

Genetic counseling is done by qualified professionals, usually found at university medical centers and hospitals. Counselors can guide you through the testing process to assure appropriate testing is selected. They will help with the understanding of the test results and an understanding of the disease.(5) Counseling can help with decisions that will need to be made regarding treatment and work with clinicians to help patients and their families understand the progression of the disease. They can help educate regarding risk and assist in making procreation decisions. (6)

Additional Resources

- Information about genetic counseling and genetic testing can be found at: Genetics Home Reference >> Handbook >> Genetic Consultation or >>Genetic Testing. **www.ghr.nlm.nih.gov/handbook/consult**.
- Additional information about genetic counseling and locating a genetic counselor in your area or state can be found at the website: National Society of Genetic Counselors >> Find a Genetic Counselor. **www.nsgc.org**.

Retinitis Pigmentosa

Retinitis pigmentosa (RP) is the most common of the retinal dystrophies. People with RP have photoreceptors that are programmed for early degeneration and death. It is typically called a rod-cone dystrophy, because the photoreceptors that are most affected are the neurons called rods. Rods are sensitive to low light levels and motion. They are responsible for our ability to adapt to seeing in dim light and awareness of our side vision. Loss of rods means loss of night vision and visual field.

RP can appear as a stand-alone eye disease, or it can be part of a syndrome, that affects the eyes along with other parts of the body.

Genetics

The genetics of RP are complex. The gene mutation can be multiple and varied. Even the presentation, progression, age of onset, and severity are variable. Much research is ongoing to understand the links between the various gene mutations and how it manifests as RP.

There are three different genetic inheritance patterns. The clinical presentation and the visual impact may be similar. But even within each of these three groups, there are subgroups of the disease based on which gene or groups of genes are mutated.

The description of each group below is very general.

1. Autosomal Dominant RP.
   - Mildest form;
   - Later in life onset of signs and symptoms;
   - Maintains central vision and better visual acuity to a later stage of life; and
   - Clear family inheritance pattern.
2. Autosomal Recessive RP.

- Slightly different clinical presentation than autosomal dominant RP;
- A more rapid loss of visual function;
- Variable severity and prognosis; and
- No other family members may be affected.

3. X-Linked RP.
   - Most severe of the three inheritance patterns for loss of visual function and visual acuity;
   - Affects children at a young age with night blindness;
   - Abnormalities of light adaption can be detected in carriers of x- linked RP (unaffected parents and siblings); and
   - Does affect both males and females.(7)

Signs and Symptoms

The first symptom is night blindness (nyctalopia). The perception is of not being able to see in dim light or the incapability to adjust to changing light levels. Adaption to different light levels becomes more difficult, and bright light can dazzle with uncomfortable glare. Someone with RP may have difficulty moving through dimly lit areas and driving at dusk.

The progressive loss of the light and motion sensitive rod neurons of the peripheral vision results not only in night blindness, but also the development of visual field defects. Visual field loss may not be noticed initially, as one eye may compensate for the loss of visual field of the other eye. Overall, however, the loss of visual function is in both eyes, fairly equally. There have been antidotal reports of people with RP seeing light flashes or shimmering lights.(7)

The visual field loss is a concentric constriction, meaning the visual field narrows left, right, up, and down, making the visual field smaller over time. By the fourth and fifth decade of life, the visual field loss can be significant enough to affect mobility. Someone with RP may find themselves bumping into furniture, doorways, or not seeing cars in their side vision. Enough visual field may be lost to render tunnel vision. That is vision comparable to living life looking through a keyhole.

Other visual function losses can include changes in color perception, especially in the blue range. Loss of color vision is more likely in those with poor central vision.(8) Cataracts are also prevalent in RP, (about 50%), particularly the type called posterior sub-capsular cataracts.(9) Late stage RP can result in loss of the central neurons of the macula, called cones, which can result in blindness. The odds are that someone with RP, will retain some central vision.(10)

Management

1. Nutritional Supplements. High doses of vitamin A in combination with fish oils (DHA) have been proposed to slow the progression of the retinal degeneration. One study indicated that this combination of vitamin A and a diet rich in omega 3 fish oils "should make it possible for many patients with typical retinitis pigmentosa to retain both visual acuity and central visual field

for most of their lives."(11) However another study evaluating previous trials, indicated that the use of vitamin A and fish oils to slow progression of visual field loss, photoreceptor responsiveness, and visual acuity loss, are questionable.(12) The benefit of high-dose vitamin A must be considered against its liver toxicity. There have been several studies, including the AREDS, which is a study that evaluated the benefits of nutrients for the macula, suggest that omega 3 fatty acids are beneficial for photoreceptor health.

2. <u>Sunglasses and Tinted Eyewear</u>. Tinted eyewear is helpful to increase contrast, reduce glare from sunlight, and reduce scatter for those with cataracts. Sunglasses are essential for protection. Although the use of tinted eyewear to eliminate exposure to UV light has not proven as a means to decrease the progression of RP(13), increased exposure to UV and high energy blue light can speed up the progression of retinal degeneration.(7)

3. <u>Assistive Technology</u>. Magnifiers are not as effective for those with peripheral field loss. However, those electronic devices or computer screens that have the ability to change color polarity, for example, white or yellow print against black, may be helpful for reducing glare to increase comfort when reading.

4. <u>Adequate Indoor Lighting and Portable Light Sources</u>. There should be adequate task lighting for work areas. Reading lamps should be over the shoulder, directed at the reading material. Lights that are mounted on the eyeglass frame and directed at

the work area can be purchased. Having on hand a light source for dimly lit situations can be helpful. Small LED flashlights, like those that can be attached to key chains can be helpful in dim walkways or hallways. The very small magnifiers that have an LED light can be used in restaurants and theaters. The benefit of the small video magnifiers, is not their capability to magnify, but the ability to change polarity to reduce glare off of reading material.

5. Specialty Aids for Field Enhancement. Although nothing can completely replace the loss of visual field, lens add-ons like Fresnel prisms and mirrors can be placed on the glasses, in the area of field loss, to give enhanced access to viewing objects in the area of vision loss.

6. Field Expanders. These devices may help in the later stages of the disease for those that have severely restricted visual fields. Field expanders are devices, such as telescopes used in reverse. This has the effect of increasing the field of view, but consequently makes objects appear smaller and details may be lost.

   Both field enhancers and field expanders need to be prescribed and fitted by a low vision professional. Remember, nothing can take the place of lost visual field. These aids are used intermittently and briefly to access the environment. There will be some training and adaption required.

7. Rehabilitation Services. Therapists can help with adaption.

Techniques of visual scanning, in which a pattern of eye movements are used to evaluate the environment can be learned. Orientation and Mobility Specialists can also help with mobility training for those who have lost the ability to navigate their surroundings because of severe visual field loss.

8. Counseling. RP patients need to understand the disease process and can benefit from counseling to help them with the psycho-social aspect of dealing with a progressive, potentially blinding disease process. Counselors can help with education and job-related decision making. They can also help with the understanding of the genetics of RP to assist in decisions of procreation.

9. Biotechnology. Presently, RP is one of the hereditary diseases for which stem cell therapy, gene replacement therapy, and retinal prosthesis studies are being conducted.

Additional reading:

- Telander, David G., Roy Hampton Sr., et al. RP Clinical Presentation. Medscape. Age-Related Eye Disease Study 2. (AREDS2). **www.nei.nih.gov/areds2/**
- Understanding Retinitis pigmentosa. (PDF). Kellogg Eye Center, University of Michigan. **www.kellogg.umich.edu/.../Understand-Retinitis-pigmentosa.pdf**.
- Learning About Retinitis Pigmentosa. National Human Genome Research Institute. **https://www.genome.gov**/

Choroideremia

Choroideremia is a progressive, degenerative disease of the choroid and retinal pigment epithelium (RPE). The choroid is the vascular bed of tiny blood vessels that bring oxygen and nutrients to the RPE, photoreceptors, and neurons of the retina.

The disease is due to a non-functioning protein, called the Rab-1 escort protein that is the result of a mutation of the CHM gene. Without this protein, the blood vessels of the choroid and the RPE degenerate and die. Without the choroid and RPE, death of the essential neuro-sensory retina follows. It is thought that there are several different mutations involving the Rab-1 protein that may explain the variability of age of onset, severity, and progression of the disease, even within affected families.(14)

This inherited disease can be misdiagnosed, at least initially, as retinitis pigmentosa, or as one of two other peripheral retinal diseases; gyrate atrophy and inherited choroidal atrophy.(15)

Genetics

Choroideremia has an x-linked recessive hereditary pattern, and usually runs in families. The X chromosome is one of the sex determining chromosomes. Males have one x chromosome (XY), and females have two X chromosomes (XX). The CHM gene mutation is on the X chromosome. The males with their one X chromosome and the mutation will have the disease. Females who have the mutation on one X chromosome, and have a normal second X chromosome, will not have the disease. They are termed carriers. It is possible however, for a female to develop the disease, if both parents are carriers, and she gets two X chromosomes with the mutation.

The X-linked recessive inheritance pattern means that the sons of a carrier mother have a 50 percent chance of having the disease. The daughters of a carrier mother have a 50 percent chance of being carriers. The sons of a father, who has the disease, will not have sons with the disease, but all of his daughters will be carriers.

Signs and Symptoms

Similar to the other retinal dystrophies, one of the first signs is difficulty with adapting to dim or dark lighting, and impaired night vision ("night blindness"). This usually occurs in the first and second decades of life. The progression is slow and variable. The first signs of retinal changes may occur as early as three years old.(16) What the doctor sees is areas of pigment stippling (dots and specks), and areas that are lighter in color. These are areas of retinal pigment cell loss. Visual field loss occurs next, in a ring-like 'blind' area. If you were to think of the eye ball as a globe, the concentric ring would be at the 'equator'. Over time this area expands and works its way towards the central vision area. The result will be 'tunnel vision', similar to looking through a keyhole. This usually occurs in a person's 20s and 30s. Up until age 40, good central vision may be maintained. A study by Roberts et al., in 2002, reported that 89 percent of participants below age 60 had visual acuity of 20/50 or better. There was a decline in vision to 20/200 or worse for 33percent of those over the age of 60.(17)

Carrier females, who do not exhibit the full blown disease of choroideremia, can show signs to a much lesser degree, revealing their carrier status. They may experience problems with dark adaption and exhibit patchy chorio-retinal degeneration. (18)

Management

1. Sunglasses and Tinted Eyewear. Tinted eyewear is helpful to increase contrast, reduce glare from sunlight, and reduce scatter for those with cataracts. Sun wear should always be worn for protection. The use of tinted eyewear to reduce exposure to UV light has not proven as a means to decrease the progression of choroiderema. (7)

2. Assistive Technology. Magnifiers are not as effective for those with peripheral field loss. However, those electronic devices or computer screens that have the capability to change color polarity, for example, white or yellow print against black, may be helpful for reducing glare to increase comfort when reading.

3. Adequate Indoor Lighting and Portable Light Sources. There should be adequate task lighting for work areas. Reading lamps should be over the shoulder, directed at the reading material. Lights that are mounted on the eyeglass frame and directed at the work area can be purchased. Having on hand a light source for dimly lit situations can be helpful. Small LED flashlights, like those that can be attached to key chains can be helpful in dim walkways or hallways. The very small magnifiers that have an LED light can be used in restaurants and theaters. The benefit

of the small video magnifiers, is not their capability to magnify, but the ability to change polarity to reduce glare off of reading material.

4. Specialty Aids for Field Enhancement. Although nothing can completely replace the loss of visual field, lens add-ons like Fresnel prisms and mirrors can be placed on the glasses, in the area of field loss, to give an enhanced access to viewing objects in the area of vision loss.

5. Field Expanders. These devices may help in the later stages of the disease for those that have severely restricted visual fields. Field expanders are devices such as telescopes used in reverse. This has the effect of increasing the field of view, but consequently makes objects appear smaller and details may be lost.

   Both field enhancers and field expanders need to be prescribed and fitted by a low vision professional. Remember, nothing can take the place of lost visual field. These aids are used intermittently and briefly to access the environment. There will be some training and adaption required.

6. Rehabilitation services. Therapists can help with adaption. Techniques of visual scanning, in which a pattern of eye movements are used to evaluate the environment can be learned. Orientation and Mobility Specialists can also help with mobility training for those who have lost the capability to navigate their surroundings because of severe visual field loss.

7. Counseling. Choroideremia patients need to understand the disease process and can benefit from counseling to help them with the psycho-social aspects of dealing with a progressive, potentially blinding, disease process. Counselors can help with educational and job related decision making. They can also help with the understanding of the genetics of choroideremia to help in decisions of procreation.

8. Biotechnology. Gene replacement therapy and stem cell therapy, at this time, has the potential to treat choroideremia. There have been some successful clinical trials of gene therapy for Choroideremia, but is not yet available to those outside the research facility.

Additional Reading:

- Genetics Home Reference >>Conditions >>Choroideremia **http://ghr.nlm.nih.gov/condition/choroideremia**
- Choroideremia Research Foundation **http://choroideremia.org/**

The Macular Dystrophies:

Stargardt's Disease and Best's Disease

Stargardt's Disease (Stargardt's Macular Dystrophy)

Stargardt's Disease is an autosomal recessive genetic mutation, know as a cone dystrophy. In 1997, the defective gene responsible for Stargardt's disease was identified. Since then, 19 mutations of this gene have been identified.(19) The various mutations of the gene causing Stargardt's disease results in differences in severity, age of onset, and progression of disease.

The gene is the ABCA4 gene. (Referred to as the ABCR gene in older literature.) This gene makes a protein essential in the biochemical light sensing cycle of the cone neurons. It is the failure of this protein to function which results in the buildup of toxins. The toxins kill off the very important support cells for the cone neurons, called the retinal pigment epithelium (RPE). Death of the RPE, with the accumulation of toxins, results in a by-product called lipofuscin. Lipofuscin deposits are the hallmark of Stargardt's disease. These flecks of lipofuscin are described as fish-tail shaped, comma-shaped, or crescent-shaped.

Genetics

Typical Stargardt's disease has an autosomal recessive inheritance pattern. This means that both parents must be carriers of the defective gene, but may be unaffected. Each child born to this couple has a 25 percent chance of having the disease. Stargardt's diseases can be described as 4 basic types, based on severity, age of onset, and progression. The end result, however, is very similar. There is the loss of the central vision area with moderate to marked decrease in visual acuity.

1. Stargardt's Disease Type I, also known as Juvenile Hereditary Macular Dystrophy.
   - age of onset is 8 to 12 years old;
   - autosomal recessive, most likely no known other family members affected (except possible siblings);
   - affects both sexes equally; and
   - decrease in visual acuity can be rapid.
2. Stargardt's Disease Type II, aka. Late-Onset or Adult-Onset Stargardt's Disease
   - autosomal recessive, with no prior family history;
   - older age of onset, 20s or 30s;
   - a milder ABCA4 mutation;
   - vision loss is gradual; and
   - fairly good visual acuity may be maintained into 30s or 40s.
3. Fundus flavimaculatus
   - macula is less affected;
   - better visual outcome;
   - retinal findings similar to Stargardt's flecks;

- maybe asymptomatic; and
- thought to be the result of a very mild ABCA4 mutation.

4. Autosomal Dominant Stargardt's Disease
   - other genes have been identified as responsible for this macular dystrophy, therefore it is referred to as a Stargardt-like disease.
   - rare;
   - clear hereditary pattern, in which other family members are affected; and
   - similar retinal and macular presentation to fundus flavimaculatus and Stargardt's disease. (20)

Signs and Symptoms

The first sign an examining doctor may see are the comma-shaped flecks of lipofuscin surrounding the central vision areas. These flecks are yellowish and retractile. Initially, these flecks may not have any impact on vision.

The first symptom a person with Stargardt's disease might notice is a ring scotoma. The central vision is fine, maybe even 20/20, and the side vision is good, but there is this area, just outside the central vision, that is a blind ring. Reading time will slow down, letters on signs may disappear, and small moving objects may seem to disappear, then jump back into vision.

Another symptom is light sensitivity, seemingly more so than 'normal' individuals. There will be discomfort to the eyes when confronted with sunlight, bright lights, or flashing lights. The capability to adapt to dark or dim light is diminished after exposure to bright sunlight.

Over time the flecks become more numerous, the ring gets larger and appears to be moving inward to the central vision. The cone neurons in this area are degenerating and dying. Light flashes may be evident. In the end there will be a loss of visual acuity. The larger the area of vision loss, the poorer the outcome for visual acuity will be. Color vision may be affected in the late stages, particularly in the red and greens. (21)

Here is the good news. Although the critical central vision is lost, those afflicted with Stargardt's do not go 'blind' in the sense that there is no useable vision. Visual acuity may decrease to the legal designation of blind, which is set at 20/200. Even so, those with Stargardt's, like others with macular disease, have the rest of the retina to learn to use effectively. Learning to use an alternative location to view with is called eccentric fixation. (See chapter on Adaptive Techniques.) The vision of eccentric fixation will never be as good as the macular vision, but learning techniques of adaption becomes the 'norm.'

Management

1. Magnification. Those with Stargardt's disease do very well with magnification. Life becomes a quest to make it all larger. Telescopes and bioptic lenses help with distance viewing to bring images closer, and make them larger. High plus glasses, magnifiers, large print, and assistive technology can be of great help towards leading a 'normal' life.

2. Sunglasses and Tinted Eyewear. Protection against UV light exposure is important. Toxic waste products build up secondary to light exposure, and UV is the most damaging. Sunglasses should always be worn outside, even on overcast days.

3. Nutritional Supplements. Antioxidants as a group have been proposed as beneficial for those with eye disease. Antioxidants, lutein and zeaxanthin are dietary supplements included in the AREDS 2 (stands for Age Related Eye Disease Study).(22) Although Stargardt's was not specifically evaluated with the macular degeneration formula, others are researching the possible benefits to slow the progression of SD. DHA, which is an omega 3 fatty acid, has also been studied as a means to improve retinal function and to slow the progression of SD.(23)

   Stargardt's patients should avoid vitamin A and beta-carotene, as it is the waste products of vitamin A metabolism that is in the toxic yellow flecks.

4. Rehabilitative Services. Often because of the slow progression of the disease, which occurs simultaneously in both eyes, the Stargardt's patient will often learn eccentric viewing on their own as an adaptive technique. Others can be taught the technique of eccentric viewing by an optometrist or low vision therapist.

5. Biotechnology. Stargardt's disease is presently one of the hereditary eye diseases for which gene replacement therapy and stem cell therapy is actively being studied.

Additional Reading:

- Understanding Stargardt's Disease. Kellogg Eye Center, University of Michigan. **www.kellogg.umich.edu/patientcare/downloads/Understanding-Stargardt.pdf**
- Age-Related Eye Disease Study 2. (AREDS2) **www.nei.nih.gov/areds2/**

Best's Disease

(Vitelliform Macular Dystrophy, BVMD)

Best's Disease is a rare, autosomal dominant disorder of a retinal pigment epithelial cell protein (protein called bestrophin). It is called vitelliform because of the appearance of yellow, centrally located deposits. To an examining doctor, the central lesion looks like an egg yolk, because it is round, yellow, and can be slightly raised. These deposits are a result of retinal pigment epithelium dysfunction, which leaves behind the waste product lipofuscin. It is this build up of toxic waste products that results in the death of the retinal pigment epithelium, and the light-sensitive photoreceptor cells above it, that depend on the retinal pigment epithelium for metabolic support. Progression of the disease is slow. There may be good visual acuity for decades, with the most devastating central vision loss after the age forty.

Genetics

The defect is of the VMD2 gene.(24) The autosomal dominant pattern of inheritance means that if only one parent has the gene, each child born to that couple has a 50 percent chance of inheriting the disease. Because it is autosomal dominant, it tends to run in families.

Signs and Symptoms

Best's disease varies by how it is expressed, by age of onset, clinical findings, progression, and final outcome.(25)

Studies of Best's Disease describe it as having 5 stages: (26, 27, 28)

Stage 1: Pre-vitelliform Stage. There is normal visual acuity with very subtle central macular changes. Usually this occurs in the first decade of life. Best's disease can be identified as early as 3 to 5 years old.

Stage 2: The Vitelliform Stage. The macular change is more evident with a raised, yellow lesion, described as having an 'egg yolk appearance.' Vision may still be good. The Vitelliform Stage usually occurs in the first to second decade of life. Late in this stage the macula may be described as having a 'scrambled egg appearance.'

Stage 3: The Pseudohypopyon Stage. Pseudohypopyon means a development of an area of fluid. There is some leakage of the yellow deposits into the area just beneath the retina. The first symptom may be some blurring with distortion of images. Visual acuity drops to 20/40 or 20/50. This is likely to happen in the second decade of life.

Stage 4: The Atrophic Stage. Decades have passed and the central vision area has suffered damage secondary to waste accumulation, leakage, and as a consequence may have developed the abnormal growth of the very fragile, leaky blood vessels in a process called neovascularization. In the central vision area, the retinal pigment epithelial cells and the photoreceptor cells that dependent on them, have died and degenerated, leaving a visible scar. Vision drops to 20/200 or 20/400. This stage occurs later in life, most commonly over the age of 40.

There is some variability in expression and progression.

Testing for Best's Disease

The hallmark tests for Best's disease are an electrooculography (EOG) and electroretinography (ERG). These two tests are usually done in a referral center that does specialized testing. While the ERG should be normal, it is the EOG which will give low abnormal results, thus differentiating it from other macular dystrophies.(29) Visual acuity and the Amsler grid should be monitored for progression.

Management

Any treatment for Best's Disease will not cure or prevent the various stages of the disease, but will attempt to slow the progression.

1. Magnifiers. The best aids are magnification for near, in the form of high plus reading glasses and magnifiers. Telescopes and bioptic lenses help with distance viewing to bring images closer, and make them larger.

2. Sunglasses and Tinted Lenses. Protective eyewear should be worn to decrease the effects of UV light damage.

3. Regular Eye Exams. The central macular area should be monitored for the formation of the sub-retinal neovascularization, especially in the later stages. If these abnormal blood vessels are seen, the doctor will opt to give a laser treatment to stem the growth and/or inject anti-VEGF medication to preserve the remaining vision.

4. Nutritional Supplements. Anti-oxidant supplements, along with a healthy nutritional diet, have been recommended to stabilize the progression of age-related macular degeneration. Although Bests disease was not a part of the Age-Related Eye Disease Study (AREDS 2), those with BVMD may benefit from the anti-oxidants, lutein, zeaxanthin, and DHA supplement formula developed through the study of patients with age-related macular degeneration.

5. Rehabilitative Services. Best's disease patients do not go blind, but will lose the central macular vision area. Through rehabilitative services, eccentric fixation can be learned as an adaptive technique. Eccentric fixation helps someone with central vision loss to utilize other parts of the vision for primary viewing.

6. Counseling. Counselors can provide guidance through the diagnostic testing, help with an understanding of the progression of the disease, and help with making decisions related to work and education.,

7. Biotechnology. Best's Disease one of the inherited eye diseases

currently undergoing clinical trials for gene replacement therapy and stem cell therapy.

Additional reading:

- Vitelliform Macular Dystrophy Genetics Home Reference. **ghr.nlm.nih.gov**.
- Age-Related Eye Disease Study 2. (AREDS2). **www.nei.nih.gov/areds2/**.

Albinism

Albinism is a hereditary disorder associated with a person having an abnormally low amount of pigmentation. The name comes from the Latin word albus (or alba), meaning 'white.' Contrary to general perception, it is an inherited disorder that is variable in appearance and the degree to which it affects the individual. It turns out that there is a whole spectrum of genetic mutations, which range from severe to near normal.

The most severe form, called Oculocutaneous Albinism (OCA), is more complete, affecting hair, skin, and eyes. Ocular Albinism (OA) has milder abnormalities, hair and skin pigmentation is normal or near normal, and the abnormality predominantly affects the eyes. It is estimated that there are as many as 10 different types of oculocutaneous albinism and 4 different types of ocular albinism. (30)

Oculocutaneous Albinism (OCA)

Historically, albinism was defined as 'tyrosinase-negative' and 'tyrosinase-positive.' The test for tyrosinase is done on a hair bulb. This is where hair pigment is produced for hair color. A negative test indicates that the person is negative for the enzyme tyrosinase, which is essential for pigment production. Tyrosinase-negative albinism is now known as oculocutaneous albinism 1 (OCA1). It is the most severe form. This is but one form of OCA.

Within the tyrosinase-positive group, there are many other pigment producing defects, which are due to other proteins involved in melanin (pigment) production or transport. This means that someone can have the tyrosinase enzyme and still have oculocutaneous albinism. These other oculocutaneous, tyrosinase-positive defects are identified by numbers: OCA2, OCA3, and OCA4. Each of these varies by the amount of pigment produced, which can accumulate over a lifetime, accounting for the differences in appearance among those with albinism.(31) Tyrosinase-negative OCA1 and tyrosinase-positive OCA2 are the two most commonly inherited forms of albinism. (32)

There are also forms of albinism associated with syndromes. These diseases have other systemic health issues combined with albinism traits:

- Chediak-Higashi Syndrome: OCA pigment abnormalities, abnormal bleeding, and a susceptibility to infection.
- Hermansky-Pudlak Syndrome: OCA, bleeding abnormalities, and lipid storage disease.

- Griscelli Syndrome: Hypo pigmentation, silver hair, intellectual disabilities, seizures (type 1), or recurrent infections (type 2).
- Waardenburg Syndrome: Pigment abnormalities, eyelid and facial abnormalities and deafness.

Ocular Albinism (OA)

While OCA involves eye, skin, and hair, ocular albinism (OA) involves primarily the eyes. Skin and hair can be normal or near normal. Ocular symptoms are variable, and are dependent on the amount of pigment present. The more pigment, the better the visual function. While visual acuity of someone with OCA may range from 20/80 to 20/400, someone with OA may have better visual acuity in the range of 20/25 to 20/300. (33)

Genetics

Oculocutaneous albinism (OCA) has an autosomal recessive inheritance pattern. That means that both parents have to have the gene, and each child born to that couple has a 25 percent chance of inheriting OCA.

The more severe form, OCA1, indicates a defect in the TYR-1gene. This genetic defect does not allow for any pigment production. The other tyrosinase positive forms of OCA (OCA 2, 3, and 4) have other genetic defects of tyrosinase associated proteins or transport proteins. The differences in gene mutation account for the variability in the capability to produce some pigment.

Ocular albinism (OA) has a sex-linked X chromosome inheritance pattern. This means ocular albinism is passed to male offspring by way of their single X chromosome. If the father has OA, and the mother is not a carrier, none of his sons will develop OA, but all of his daughters will be carriers. If the mother is a carrier, and the father is not, there is a 50 percent chance her sons will have OA and 50 percent chance her daughters will be carriers.

There is great variability among female carriers as to whether or not they exhibit any signs. Female carriers may have very light eye pigmentation, and possibly poor visual acuity and nystagmus.(34)

Signs and Symptoms

All forms of albinism affect the eyes. This discussion of albinism will focus on the ocular abnormalities. The eye problems encountered by those with albinism are:

1. Decreased visual acuity;
2. Nystagmus (repetitive eye movement);
3. Strabismus (binocular vision anomaly);
4. Photophobia (light sensitivity); and
5. High refractive error.

Whether it is a genetic defect of tyrosinase, or another of the albinism genetic defects, pigment production is decreased during the early development of the eye. The pigment, called melanin, of the developing embryo is found to be produced in the skin, mucous membranes, stria vascularis of the ear, and in the eye.

The eye pigment is formed in the uveal coat, which is an outer layer of the eye, and the retinal pigment epithelium (rpe) layer within the eye. Important to the development of the eye is this RPE. Without a developing retinal pigment epithelium, overall development of the eye is slowed. The RPE is also important for the neural organization of the eye. A poorly developed rpe results in an underdeveloped central vision area called the macula, and a misrouting of the nerves that connect between the eye and the brain by way of the optic nerve.(35)

The underdeveloped macula results in poor visual acuity and nystagmus. Nystagmus is the involuntary back and forth movement of the eyes, often described as a rapid movement like a pendulum, a see-saw, or rotary motion. An eye that has not developed a central vision area takes on nystagmus. Nystagmus develops in childhood, but can become less conspicuous with age.(36)

The misrouting of the nerves of the optic nerve to the brain contributes to strabismus. Commonly, strabismus is identified as a 'lazy eye.' The eyes affected with albinism, because of the misdirected wiring of the nerves to the brain, are not working together. It takes two eyes working together to give good depth perception. Strabismus, results in a lack of depth perception.

Pigmentation of the eye is also essential for protecting the eye from UV radiation damage. The iris, which is the first line of defense, may be lightly pigmented or not pigmented at all. The iris is the colored diaphragm which gives us the color of our eyes. It opens up or closes down depending on light levels. The light-eyed albino has no protective iris pigments. Light can pass through the pale, translucent iris. Bright lights not shielded by the pigment of the iris are more intense for those with albinism, making them photophobic (light sensitive).

The retinal pigment epithelium, besides being a supporting structure for the retina, also serves to absorb light rays within the eye. Without a functional RPE, light that enters the eye is not absorbed, but bounces around. Light seems particularly bright, adding to their photophobia.

The slow, underdevelopment of the eye also contributes to high refractive errors, resulting in those with albinism as being very nearsighted, farsighted, or having a significant astigmatism. Their eyeglasses may be thicker than the average person, and still vision may not be good.

Management

Those with albinism should receive regular eye examinations. They can greatly benefit from an evaluation by a low vision specialist. They can be helped with:

1. Corrective eyewear. The first place to start is to get a set of eyeglasses that can best correct the visual acuity. It is also possible that a bifocal lens, and prisms set into the lenses, can help dampen down the nystagmus.(37)

2. Magnifiers and Assistive Technology. Those with poor central vision benefit from the magnification. . Technology is your friend. Video magnifiers and CCTV can help with reading activities. Computers, tablets, and cell phones have built-in accessibility features for those with low vision

3. Telescopes and Bioptics. Distance objects can be made to appear larger and closer through the use of lens systems. The telescope can either be hand-held, or mounted into eyeglasses. A bioptic is a small telescope mounted in a high position in the prescription lens. These are commonly prescribed for those who still qualify for driving privileges.

4. UV Light Protection. Without the pigment of skin and eyes to provide protection from the damaging effects of sunlight, it is an absolute necessity that those with pigment deficiencies wear protective sunglasses and hats with visors.

5. Rehabilitation Services. This includes mobility training. Therapists can help with adaptive techniques and the use of accessibility technology for school and work. Mobility training teaches the best techniques for travel for the more severely impaired.

6. Counseling. Counselors can help with the psychological aspects of not only dealing with the low vision aspects but also with the often social implications of albinism. Additionally, they can aid with genetic counseling and procreation decisions.

7. Biotechnology. Albinism is one of the hereditary eye diseases for which gene replacement therapy and stem cell therapy is being studied.

Additional Reading:

- Vision for Tomorrow Foundation **www.visionfortomorrow.org/albinism/**

- The National Organization for Albinism and Hypopigmentation **www.albinism.org/**

References:

1. Stone, Edwin M. MD, PhD; Genetic Testing for Inherited Eye Disease. JAMA Ophthalmology Feb. 2007, Vol. 125, No.2.
2. Genetics Home Reference >> Handbook >> Genetic Testing. Retrieved from **http://ghr.nlm.nih.gov/handbook/testing?show=all#riskslimitations**
3. Stone, Edwin M., MD, PhD et al. Recommendations for Genetic Testing for Inherited Eye Disease. Report of the American Academy of Ophthalmology Task Force for Genetic Testing.
4. Direct-to-Consumer Genetic Tests. Federal Trade Commission, Consumer Information. Retrieved from Federal Trade Commission Website. **http://www.consumer.ftc.gov/articles/0166-direct-consumer-genetic-tests**
5. Frequently Asked Questions About Genetic Counseling. Genetic Disorders, Genomics, and Healthcare. National Human Genome Research Institute Website. Retrieved from **http://www.genome.gov/19016905**
6. About Genetic counselors. National Society of Genetic Counselors website. Retrieved from **http://www.nsgc.org/**
7. Merin, S. Inherited Eye Disease, Diagnosis and Management. Taylor and Francis, 2005.
8. Fishman GA, Color vision defects in retinitis pigmentosa. Ann Ophthalmol1981;12:609-618.
9. Merin S. Cataract formation in retinitis pigmentosa. Birth Defects 198218:187-191.
10. Grover S., Fishman GA., Alexander KR., Anderson RJ., Derlacki DJ. Visual

acuity impairment in patients with retinitis pigmentosa. Ophthalmology 1996; 103:1593-1600.

11. Berson Eliot L., Rosner, Bernard, Sandberg, Michael A., Weigel-DiFranco, Carol, Willett, Walter. ω-3 Intake and Visual Acuity in Patients With Retinitis Pigmentosa Receiving Vitamin A.. Arch Ophthalmol. 2012; 130(6):707-711.

12. Rayapod S., Schwartz SG., Wang, x., Chavis P., Vitamin A and fishoils for retinitis pigmentosa. Cochrane Database Syst Rev. 2013, Dec. 19; 12.

13. Miyake Y, Sugita S, Horiguchi M, Yagasaki K: Light deprivation and retinitis pigmentosa. Am. J. Ophth. 110: 305-306, 1990.

14. Merin, S. Inherited Eye Disease, Diagnosis and Management. Taylor and Francis, 2005.482-483

15. Merin, S. Inherited Eye Disease, Diagnosis and Management. Taylor and Francis, 2005.

16. Merin, S. Inherited Eye Disease, Diagnosis and Management. Taylor and Francis, 2005.477

17. Roberts MF, Fishman GA, Roberts DK, Heckenlively JR, Weleber RG, Anderson RJ, Grover S. Retrospective, longitudinal, and cross sectional study of visual acuity impairment in choroideraemia. Br J Ophthalmol. 2002 Jun;86(6):658-62.

18. Moosajee M, Ramsden SC, Black GC, Seabra MC, Webster AR. Clinical utility gene card for: **choroideremia**. Eur J Hum Genet. 2014 Apr;22(4). doi: **10.1038/ejhg**.2013.183. Epub 2013 Aug 21.

19. AlliKmetis, Singh N, Sun H, et al. A photoreceptor cell-specific ATP binding transporter gee(ABCR) is mutated in recessive Stargardt's macular dystrophy. Nat Genet 1997,15;236-246.

20. Merin S. Inherited Macular Diseases. Inherited Eye Diseases, Diagosis and management. Taylor and Francis, 2005.

21. Merin S. Inherited Macular Diseases. Inherited Eye Diseases, Diagosis and management. Taylor and Francis, 2005. 197.

22. Age-Related Eye Disease Study 2. (AREDS2) **www.nei.nih.gov/AREDS2/** For the public; What the Age-Related Eye Disease Studies Means for You.

23. Querques, Giuseppe, Benlian, Pascale, Chanu, BErnard, Leveziel, Nicolas, Coscas, Gabriel, Soubrane, Gisele, and Soulied, Eric H. DHA supplementation for late onset Stargardt disease: NAT-3 study Clin Ophthalmol. 2010; 4: 575–580.

24. Petrukhin K, Koisu MJ, Bakall B, et al. Identification of the gene responsible for Best's macular dystrophy. Nat Genet 1998; 19:241-247.

25. Merin S. Inherited Macular Diseases. Inherited Eye Diseases, Diagosis and management. Taylor and Francis, 2005: 217.

26. Deutman AF. The Hereditary Dystrophiesof the Posterior Pole of the Eye. Asen, Netherlands:Van Gorcum, 1971.

27. Godel V, Chaine G, Reganbogen L, Coscas G. Best's Viitelliformmacular dystrophy. Acta Ophthalmol 1986;s(suppl): 11-31.

28. Mohler CW, Fine SL. Long term evaluation of patients with Best's vitelliformsustrophy. Ophthalmology 1981; 88:688-691,

29. Merin S. Inherited Macular Diseases. Inherited Eye Diseases, Diagosis and management. Taylor and Francis, 2005: 215.

30. Merin S. Albinism. Inherited Eye Diseases, Diagosis and management. Taylor and Francis, 2005: 215.

31. Oetting WS. Brillant MH. King RA. The clinical spectrum of albinism in humans. Molecular Medicine Today: 1996l(2)8.

32. Merin S. Albinism. Inherited Eye Diseases, Diagosis and management. Taylor and Francis, 2005: 729.

33. Handbook of Ocular Disease. Review of Optometry. **http://cms.revoptom.com/handbook/sect58a.htm**
34. **FallsHP.Sex**-linked ocular albinismdisplaying typical fundus changesin female heterozygote. Am J Ophthalmol 1951; 34:41-50.
35. Handbook of Ocular Disease. Review of Optometry. **http://cms.revoptom.com/handbook/sect58a.htm**
36. Kriss A, Russell-Eggitt I, Harris CM, Lloyd IC, Taylor D. Aspects of Albinism. Ophthalmic Paediatric Genet. 1992;13(2):89-100.
37. Nowakowski RW. Primary Low Vision Care. Appleton and Lange, 1994.

CHAPTER 11

Clinical Research for Eye Diseases

Clinical Trials

Much of what we know about the treatment of inherited eye diseases is presently tested and researched through clinical trials. Clinical trials are the human phase of drug or treatment testing. They come after the test tube, petri dish, and/or animal studies have been completed and the preliminary results show promise in the treatment of human disease.

Clinical trials include drug tests, procedures, or therapies that are conducted by research teams that include researchers with doctorates, doctors who are researchers, technical medical support staff, and of course, administrators. Most commonly these clinical trials are conducted at centers that have research capabilities and are most often specialized medical centers, hospitals, and university medical settings.

Once it has been determined that a drug, procedure, or treatment has been proven to be effective in the laboratory, the decision to conduct clinical trials is made. Clinical trials have protocols, or well-defined plans, regarding how the testing will be conducted.. The research team determines and documents the goals of the study, research methods, materials, procedures, and the length of the study. Additionally, test subjects are selected who meet established inclusion and exclusion criteria. Who is chosen to participate depends upon factors, including: age, disease status, and general health, and the criteria (inclusion and exclusion) will vary by study. Those included in the trial are determined by the research team as the population to best support the goals of the study.

Participation in a clinical trial is voluntary. The researchers must be open and informative with the participants of any risks associated with the study. A written consent form outlines the plan, risks, and length of the study. Research team members should be available to answer any questions and concerns of the participant and their families. The decision to be a participant in a study should include, not only the patient, but should also have the support of the patient's family members.

There are very strict protocols regarding ethics and risks when conducting human clinical trials. Clinical studies in the United States must be approved and monitored by an Institutional Review Board (IRB) and the U.S. Food and Drug Administration (FDA). These governing organizations monitor the studies to be sure there is a balance of risk-to-benefit for the participants and also to protect their rights.

The benefits of being a research study participant are:

1. Access to cutting edge medical and research that should specifically help treat your disease;

2. Access to some of the most knowledgeable medical and research professionals in the disease study area;.
3. Being the proverbial guinea pig and putting yourself out there to help others in the future who will be diagnosed with the same disease; and
4. Possibly gaining the benefit of an effective treatment for your disease.

The risks of participating in clinical trials are:

1. The Great Unknown. Although medical research may have been previously performed on animal subjects, the safety and the potential for side effects is the great unknown. This is the subject and purpose of the clinical trial.
2. Time and Travel. If the research center is a distance away, consider the time it takes to get there and travel-related expense. Most research projects require patients to return many times over months and perhaps years. Testing performed on research subjects may be extensive and time consuming, involving hours spent in examination and waiting rooms, followed by a barrage of tests, and a parade of researchers.
3. Cost. The clinical trials administrators will help determine if the patient's health insurance will cover the costs of the testing and treatments. Expenses incurred by a participant and their families varies by the type of research, treatment status, and the individual's health insurance coverage.

4. No Promises. The purpose of the clinical trial is discovery. Often the researchers have an expectation of the treatment's results and have determined a favorable benefit-to-risk for the individual patient. But remember, there are no guarantees.

Clinical Phases

Clinical trials are done in a step-wise manner called phases. The phases describe where the research is at, in terms of increasing dosages and increasing the number of participants selected for the study. Each phase is dependent upon the success of the previous phase. There are four phases to a clinical trial:

Phase I. Safety. The test group selected is small, and drug dosages or the test treatments are also small. The researchers are looking for potential side effects that impact a patient negatively, and they are continuously assessing the risks to humans.

Phase II. Efficacy. Phase I has shown no, or insignificant, side effects and low risk. During Phase II,, researchers will engage more test subjects and adjust drug dosages or treatments to evaluate the effect and gauge the benefits.

Phase III. Expansion. Phase I and II are completed, and the researchers have determined that the drug or treatment is effectives and has a favorable benefit-to-risk for the treatment of the disease. A larger group of subjects are enlisted during Phase III, to confirm the effectiveness of the drug or treatment. The safety and the risk for side effects are still carefully monitored.

Phase IV Completion. The clinical trial is completed, and now the drug or treatment is open to the marketplace. Researchers turn their attention to gathering information on the drug or treatment's effectiveness, the potential for side effects in other populations, and the implications of long-term use of the drug or treatment.

Additional Reading:

- For more information about clinical trials visit : **https://clinicaltrials.gov/**. On this webpage click on: About Clinical Studies >> Learn about Clinical Studies
- At this site you can also search current and past clinical trials by topic of interest. (ex: glaucoma, retinitis pigmentosa, ocular albinism)

Gene Therapy

Gene therapy is a very active area of research that holds the potential to prevent, modify, or cure inherited diseases in the future.

Researchers are discovering and developing techniques to introduce a normal gene in place of the faulty gene in persons with genetic code variations (called mutations). The strategies of gene therapy are either to replace the defective gene, inactivate them, or introduce to the cell a new gene to diminish the effects of the disease that is caused by the defective gene. (1)

Gene therapy is a treatment technique that has been in the works for decades. The first successful gene therapy was performed in 1990 on a little girl who had the ADA enzyme deficient form of Severe Combined Immunodeficiency (SCID). Children born with this disease lack the gene which makes the enzyme (ADA). Without this enzyme, immune cells are made ineffective by the accumulation of toxins. The gene therapy was successful after multiple treatments over a period of years. She went on to live a normal, healthy life.

Since the little girl's treatment was successful, nearly a decade later, 20 other children also received gene therapy for another form of SCID, called X-linked SCID. This form is more commonly known as the 'bubble boy' disease where individuals need to live isolated in a germ-free environment. Unfortunately for them and the progress of gene therapy, five of the children went on to develop leukemia as a result of a problem with the vector selected.(2) The treatment of SCID is an indicator of how gene therapy research has evolved; there have been successes and morbid failures.

Fast forward to 2008 and The Children's hospital of Philadelphia's first successful gene therapy treatment for an inherited eye disease at. This time it was an eight-year old boy who was diagnosed with Leber's Congenital Amaurosis (LCA), an autosomal recessive disease that causes severe vision loss in the first decade of life. Through gene therapy, this little boy and several other children were able to gain back some modest, useable vision with negative effects. (3)

The Forever Fix, Gene Therapy and The Boy Who Saved It, author Ricki Lewis, details the history and the research accomplished that culminated in the successful treatment of the little boy.

Gene Therapy Basics

The genes are segments of deoxyribonucleic acid (DNA), that code for proteins made in the human cell. 'Readers' inside cells use the code to make proteins. Disease occurs because the gene code is incorrect. The result can be that:

1. An ineffective protein is made,
2. No protein is made; or
3. Too much protein is made. (4,6)

In gene therapy a new gene segment is inserted into the target cell by way of a vector. Once inside the cell, the new gene goes to work in one of several modes of action, which include:

1. The gene segment can turn "on" to give new instructions to the 'readers' in the cell for the production of the correct protein; or
2. This new gene can produce a new protein, or
3. The new gene segment is inserted to turn off a defective gene.(4)

Once the defective gene is identified, the replacement gene is engineered, and the target cells are determined, the problem becomes: How to get the therapeutic genetic material into the targeted cells? The solution depends upon the gene type, and the target cells.

Researchers are looking at various ways of getting the new genes into the target cells. The most frequently used technique is by way of a virus. Viruses, which we associate with being purveyors of disease, actually become the partners of gene therapy research. This is because of their capability to infect cells. The genetic material of the virus is removed, and the human replacement gene is packaged into the virus. (4) Viruses are the vectors. They are the vehicle which carries the gene therapy to the target cells, and do what they naturally do best, which is to infect cells. But now the infection is intentional and created by the researchers. It is a technique that will benefit the patient, and not cause disease.

Other non-viral vector techniques use other vehicles to deliver new genes to target cells. These include: liposomes (like fat globules), plasmids (independent circle of molecular DNA), stem cells (undifferentiated cells), and artificial viruses called virosomes.(1) These techniques have less safety concerns, but are less effective.(5)

This is a simplified explanation of gene therapy. The gene selection, mode of action of that gene, targeted cells, and the vector will vary by disease. Each gene therapy procedure needs to be customized.

Limitations of Gene Therapy

Through decades of research, trial and error, gene therapy is still very much under development. Several factors stand in the way of making gene therapy available to those who would benefit from the discovery of the genetic basis of disease and the advances in mapping the human genome.

1. Monogenic diseases vs. Complex diseases. A monogenic disease has one or sometimes two gene mutations, whose actions and

interactions are straight forward. The genetic information is more readily packaged into the vector and sent off. Complex genetic diseases may not be completely understood and may have several genetic variations and interactions, with no clear target cell. It is more difficult to develop gene therapies for complex diseases.(1)

2. Vector Issue. Researchers struggle with how to get genetic material into the target cells. The Viral vectors can cause problems by infecting the wrong cells, or by affecting the human genome negatively with what is their own gene expression. Non-viral vectors tend to be less efficient in targeting cells and the transfer of the genetic material.

3. Immune Reaction and Inflammatory Response. In most gene therapy research, the vector is a virus. It is possible for an individual receiving gene therapy injections, to have an immune reaction, if they have previously been exposed to the virus, and have developed an immunity. The result can be a destructive immune and inflammatory response by the patient's body.

4. Recipients Disease Status. The nature of disease is destructive. Gene therapy will not change the recipient's health status if the cells it aims to rescue are degenerated and are beyond repair. It is possible to be too late. However, gene therapy can halt a degenerative process, or cause cells that are non-functioning and undamaged to begin functioning. This is why early detection and treatment is important. (7)

5. Cost. The cost of research is high. Great strides can be made to develop customized genetic treatments for rare diseases, however, who can afford to pay for the therapy to cover the cost of research and development? Another important factor is if major pharmaceutical companies will invest funds for these treatments if the treatment population is small and the potential profitability is low? Gene therapy promises to be a cure. There may be one or several treatments over a period of time. However, unlike high cholesterol or diabetes, in which patients purchase medications on a monthly basis for the rest of their lives, gene therapy may not offer long term profitability. So ultimately the question becomes: Will gene therapy be accessible to those who need it, or will the cost be prohibitive?

6. Reproductive Concerns. There are ongoing concerns regarding how the cells of procreation (eggs and sperm) are affected. There is a danger that the vector can cross over, and affect eggs or sperm cells. This would affect future generations. Not only is this an undesired consequence, but affecting cells of reproduction is deemed unethical.(8)

Ocular Gene Therapy

Ocular gene research is being performed around the world. Ocular gene therapy accounts for only a small percentage (1.8%, n=31 at this writing) of gene therapy research. Cancer gene therapy research far exceeds all other research, including cardiovascular, neurological, inflammatory, infectious, and a host of other rarer monogenic (one gene) diseases. (9).

The eye is a unique organ. There are very specialized cells, such as photoreceptors, retinal pigment epithelium, and the optically clear cornea, which are not found anywhere else in the body. All the tissues are precisely aligned in an enclosed 'capsule' (the eyeball). These features are advantageous for treatment with gene therapy.

Because the eye has distinct cell types, viral vectors can be selected that are specific for the target cells. Whereas one viral vector may affect both photoreceptors and retinal pigment epithelium, another may affect only retinal pigment epithelium.(10) Therefore, it is easier to determine which vector is most effective.

The eye is constructed in layers of tissue, enclosed around a fluid-filled cavity. It is possible to inject the gene therapy to access a specific tissue. For example, the injection can be done below the retina (subretinal), within the retina (intraretinal), or in the fluid-filled central area (intravitreal). So the target cells can be accessed by injecting into their specific layer, which in turn acts like a compartment containing the treatment to that specific area.

Ocular gene therapy has an added benefit over other systemic gene therapies, in that the target cells are small in number. For diseases such as Severe Combined Immune-Deficiency (SCID), the targeted cells for gene therapy are those that make up the vast white blood cell system. This requires a large dose of the gene therapy and the vector by systemic infusion. In contrast, the eye is a small system, requiring a smaller dose of treatment to yield an effect.

The eye is termed "immunologically privileged",(11) meaning

immune response and inflammatory reaction within the specialized layers are suppressed within. The reaction is less likely, and will not result in a life-threatening systemic response.

There have been successes in the treatment for Leber's Congenital Amaurosis (LCA). Research is underway for other conditions such as choroideremia, retinitis pigmentosa, Stargardt's disease, neovascular macular degeneration, and glaucoma. Ocular gene therapy has the potential to halt or reverse vision loss.

Stem Cell Therapy

Stem cell therapy is familiar to most of us due to the success of bone marrow transplants and the socio-political controversy of embryonic stem cell research during the early twenty-first century. It is an established therapy that has been made new again after researchers discovered the potential of stem cells.

Bone marrow transplants for hemopoietic diseases have been performed for over thirty-plus years. It is the transfer of healthy stem cells residing in one person's bone marrow, to another person's bone marrow who has a disease of the cells of the blood system. Stem cells of the marrow are where red blood cells, white blood cells, and blood platelets are derived. This therapy has been successful in treating blood diseases such as leukemia and aplastic anemia.

In 1998, James Thomson isolated the human embryonic stem cell. Researchers have realized the potential of stem cells to help them understand disease processes and help develop replacement cell-based treatments for disease. Though incredible amounts of research are in progress, with some clinical trials, the technology is still in its early stages.

Stem Cell Basics

Stem cells are the undifferentiated cells from which all other cells of the body are derived. However, there is more than one type of stem cell: There are:

1. Human embryonic stem cells;
2. Adult stem cells;
3. Pluripotent stem cells derived from adult stem cells; and
4. Fetal stem cells.

Human Embryonic Stem Cells (hESC)

When a human egg and sperm join, their strands of DNA are paired to make a completely new genes in a single cell. The DNA inside the cell now contains all the necessary information to create a full human being, the egg-sperm combination begins to divide. When dividing the cell count doubles each time, 2 to 4 to 8 to 16 to 32 ....etc. After 4 to 5 days of dividing, a small ball of cells is formed, called a blastocyst. The central mass of the ball is the least differentiated(12); there are no nerves, skin, heart, etc. The cells are called embryonic stem cells. They have terrific potential to become whatever cell the DNA program determines them to be. The technical term is pluri (many)- potent (potential). It is during this blsatocyst stage when embryonic stem cells are harvested for embryonic stem cell research.

Stem cells can be grown in a medium to create a culture of identical stem cells. This process can be repeated for years to maintain a cell line from that original embryonic stem cell. That is one of the benefits of the embryonic stem cell; these cells can then be frozen and retrieved later when needed.

Adult Stem Cells (Tissue Stem Cells)

There are other stem cells found in the fully-formed human body, called adult stem cells. The stem cells of the bone marrow are the most familiar, but other tissues have stem cells, including the gut, heart, brain, skin, liver, cornea, and retina. They are small in number, and remain dormant until they are needed to generate repair to the tissue.(13) These cells have the potential to begin dividing and differentiating within the tissue where they are located. But these stem cells differ from embryonic stem cells, as they are committed to making cells of the tissue in which they are found, and are more difficult to isolate and grow in cell cultures. (13) The bone marrow stem cells make blood system cells, however they cannot make bone, nerves or other cells of the body. Brain stem cells can only make neurons and the supporting cells of the nervous system.

These adult stem cells offer a significant advantage as when they are harvested from an individual in need of a tissue transplant, they are recognized by the recipient's body and do not cause an immune response. Researchers are evaluating these adult stem cells as a therapy to replace damaged and destroyed tissues and organs.(13)

Stem Cells Derived from Fully Differentiated Adult Cells

There are presently, two types of adult stem cells derived from pluripotent stem cells. They are; (1). induced pluripotent stem cells (iPSC) and (2) stimulus triggered acquisition pluripotency (STAP). These are laboratory-created stem cells that have been dedifferentiated or brought back to an embryonic stem cell stage. (12,14) They can be derived from fully-differentiated cells like skin cells.

(1). Induced Pluripotent Stem Cells (IPSC). These stem cells are created by 'reprogramming' adult cells by introducing genetic material found only in embryonic stem cells. They give instructions to revert the cells back to the undifferentiated embryonic stem cell stage. The limitation of this process is that anytime new genetic material is introduced, there is the potential for a change in cell coding in the form of mutations. (12)

(2). Stimulus Triggered Acquisition Pluripotency (STAP). The STAP cells are created by stressing the adult stem cells to revert to the dedifferentiated stage.(14) This is a newer technology.

Both of these stem cells are made from the patient's own cells and would be a customized treatment for their disease. The hope is that the knowledge gained from learning to reprogram cells will contribute to the capability to regenerate damaged tissue.(15)

Fetal Stem Cells (Cord or Placenta Stem Cells)

At the time of birth, the umbilical cord, which is attached from the baby to the placenta, is cut. The blood in the cord has been discarded or saved and used by hospital laboratories to determine the baby's blood type, should the child need treatment. Researchers have found that this umbilical cord blood is rich in fetal stem cells. Like adult bone marrow stem cells, they are committed to making blood components, red blood cells, white blood cells, and platelets. These fetal cells differ, as they have not developed the features which might illicit an immune reaction from the recipient, or in reverse, launch an attack against the recipient. They act as sort of "identity neutral cells."

Issues of Stem Cell Therapy

Stem cell science and therapy is still very much under development. Researchers are trying to understand stem cells such as to how they get their cues for differentiation, integrate into tissues, and how they function. In pursuit of this knowledge, researchers must create the technologies to study them. Each cell, each tissue, and each disease presents its own set of variables that need comprehensive study prior to mainstreaming safe and effective therapy.

Some concerns about stem cell research and therapy are:

1. Teratoma Formation. Stem cells cannot be simply introduced into tissue with the hope that new tissue is formed. Without the proper cues and instructions, the pluripotent cells can; create a ball of cells, tumor-like, within a tissue.(17) These unwanted cells

are called a teratoma, and are considered cancerous.(12) This is an unwanted side effect of improperly programmed stem cells.

2. Immune Reaction. Cells derived from embryonic stem cells can be identified as non-self by a recipient immune system and that system can launch a destructive immune response to the cell treatment. The advantage of deriving adult stem cells from the individual being treated, is that it minimizes the chances of an immune reaction. However, induced pluripotent cells may still have a risk of an immune reaction.(12)

3. Cost. This is a recurrent issue seen in gene therapy and any other customized disease treatments. After all the research, development and the high-level of technology needed to provide specialized therapy, the question remains...will it be accessible to those who need it? Stem cell therapy has the potential to treat the more common diseases like diabetes and heart disease, but will the rare 'orphan' diseases be left behind?

4. The Ethical Issue. Researchers are Sensitive to the controversy of utilizing stem cells that have the potential to be a human being. As such, researchers have developed techniques to circumvent this issue. One single embryonic stem cell can be removed without destroying or harming the blastocyst.(16) The human embryonic stem cell lines derived many years ago came from the blastocysts donated to scientific researchers from clients of in-vitro fertilization clinics. These were blastocysts that would have otherwise been destroyed, but now have carried on to

potentially help future generations. Human embryonic stem cells lines, which are longstanding, will still serve an important role in research to expand our knowledge of the human cell, and as an early step in determining the safety and efficacy of various treatments.

The concern of human cloning has also been determined internationally to be unacceptable and universally prohibited.

Additional Reading:

A very good source for further reading and videos on stem cell research is the California Stem Cell Agency website:
http://www.cirm.ca.gov/our-progress/stem-cells-therapies
California's stem Cell Agency Home >>Our Progress >> stem cell basics

Ocular Stem Cell Research

The eye is composed of highly specialized nerve cells and supporting cells not found anywhere else in the body. Eye disease ultimately destroys one or more of the specialized cells. The result is a loss of function, meaning a loss of vision. Whereas gene therapy can halt or reverse disease, the loss of tissue requires cell transplantation. Stem cells have that potential, however research is still in the early stages.

Researchers are presently working on stem cell therapies for corneal degenerations, macular degenerations, inherited retinal disease, and glaucoma. The eye has a distinctive advantage as a tissue that is immune privileged, which means that due to its location and closed structure, the immune system is less likely to see foreign tissue and react negatively. It is less likely, but not altogether impossible.

The stem cell type and the replacement cell will vary by disease. Researchers are deriving retinal pigment epithelium and photoreceptors for diseases affecting the retina, like macular degenerations and inherited retinal diseases. Corneal transplant treatments have been performed with stem cell derived corneal tissue. Glaucoma treatment is typically in the form of trabecular meshwork replacement therapy.

Clinical trials of these treatments need to evaluate not only safety and efficacy, but also the ability of the replacement tissue to integrate where it is supposed to be, and how it functions. Photoreceptors, which require neural connections, present a challenge.(15) Their connections to the neural pathways traveling to the brain are what determine their functional capabilities. Other tissue, such as the retinal pigment epithelium (a support tissue), do not need that connection to function.

Most diseases of the retina and cornea destroy more than one layer of tissue. For example, the cornea, which is the clear surface of the eye, appears to be one layer of clear tissue, but is actually five layers. Replacing the complex structures of the eye may require generating multiple cell types.

Also, researchers need to evaluate the capability of the replacement cells to persist.(16) The desired outcome is to have cells integrate, function, and remain around for a while. Studies will show if repeat replacement treatments are required, or if once replaced, the new cells will remain viable for years.

There is much that is unknown. This is not only in terms of making layers of differentiated cells, but also the factors of both cellular and molecular controls and interactions between those cells.(16)

Conclusion

Gene therapy and stem cell research offer the promise to be able to restore function or replace tissue that is dysfunctional or destroyed secondary to disease. These are new ways to address disease that were previously considered untreatable. But there is still much research to be done to fully understand the cell and human development from the genetic and molecular basis.

References:

1. Approaches to Gene Therapy. Genetic Science Learning Center, , University of Utah. Learn. Genetics. Retrieved from **www.learn.genetics.utah.com/content/genetherapy/**
2. Sheridan, G., Gene Therapy Finds its Niche. Nature Biotechnology, 29 (2),121-128, Feb. 2011.
3. Simonelli, F., Maguire, A.M., Testa, F., et al; (2009) Gene Therapy for Leber's Congenital Amaurosis Is Safe and EffectiveThrough1.5 Years After Vector Administration , Molecular Therapy, 18 (3): 643-650.
4. How does gene therapy work? National Library of Medicine, Genomic Home Reference. Retrieved from **www.ghr.nim.nih.gov/**.
5. Maguire, Albert M. and Bennett, Joan, Gene Therapy for Retinal Disease, Perelman School of Medicine. Retrieved from **www.med.upenn.edu/**
6. Gene Therapy and Genetic Engineering. The Center for Health Ethics, University of Missouri School of medicine. 25 Apr. 2013.

7. Nusinowicz, S., Ridder, W.H. III, Pang, JJ., et al. Cortical visual function in the rd12 mouse model of Leber's Congenital Amaurosis after replacement gene therapy to restore retinal function., Vision Res. 2006, 46:3926-3934.
8. International law/The Genetics and Public Policy Center, Johns Hopkins University, Berman institute of Bioethics. 2010. Retrieved from **www.dnapolicy.org/**
9. Gene Therapy Clinical Trials Worldwide >> Charts and Tables >>Indications Retrieved from **www.wiley.com/**
10. Liu, Melissa M., Tuo, Jiingsheng, Chan, Chi-Chi; Republished Review: Gene therapy for ocular diseases, National Center for Biotechnology Information. Retrieved from **WWW.ncbi.nlm.nih.gov/**
11. Bryant, Juanita S. MD, Duker, Jay S. MD, and Reichel, Elias MD, pdf Gene Therapy for Retinal Disease. Review of Ophthalmology, April5, 2012. Retrieved from **www.revophth.com**/
12. Stem Cell Basics, California's Stem Cell Agency, Retrieved from **http://www.cirm.ca.gov/our-progress/stem**-cells-therapies
13. Stem Cell Information, National Institute of Health, Home > Info Center >> Stem Cells and Diseases
14. Reversing Cell Differentiation, Stem Cells . Learn. Genetics, University of Utah, Health Sciences, Home >> Stem Cells >> Reversing Cell Differentiation . Retrieved from **www.learn.genetics.utah.edu/content/stemcells/sctoday**/
15. MacLaren, R.E., Pearson R.A. Stem cell therapy and the retina, Cambridge Ophthalmology Symposium, Eye, (2007), 21, 1352-1350.
16. Christopher Kent, Senior Editor, Stem Cell Revolution: Regenerating the Eye, Review of Ophthalmology, 9/6/2012, Retrieved from http: // **www.revophth.com/content/d/features**/i/2088/c/36434/.
17. Baker, Monica. Why hES cells make teratomas Nature Reports Stem Cells Published online: 5 March 2009.|

CHAPTER 12

Adaption Techniques

Aids for adaption are covered in other chapters. These aids include magnifiers, telescopes, electronic devices, accessible media, and lens technologies. There are a few techniques an individual can learn to address specific vision impairments. These include:

1. **Getting closer** is a technique for persons with low visual acuity.
2. **Eccentric viewing** (eccentric fixation) is used by people who have lost their central vision, but who still have usable peripheral vision.
3. **Scanning** is performed by those who have lost their peripheral vision, but who still have usable central vision.

Close Viewing

Getting closer is a form of magnification. In more technical terms, it is called relative distance magnification or approach magnification. This means that the size changes in proportion to the distance from the eye. For example, if you are viewing the letter **E** at a distance of 16 inches

(40 cm) it will double in size if you move forward 8 inches (20 cm);

E at 16 inches becomes E at 8 inches.

Do you want to make your television screen twice as big? Let's say you are sitting 8 feet away from the screen. Simply move forward 4 feet, and now you have a really big, big screen television that is twice as large. If you move closer so you are 2 feet away from the television, which is a quarter of the original distance of 8 feet, the size of the screen is 4 times as large.

In other words, size is dependent upon the viewing distance. When an object is closer, it is projected as a larger image onto your retina. This larger image is projected over more retinal neurons which gives more information to the observing brain.

Here is the caveat for people who have difficulty focusing up close; you may need glasses to help focus at the very close distances. A universal sign of aging is the need for reading glasses as we approach the age of 50. In this age group, printed material held at an average reading distance of 16 inches (40 cm) appears out of focus. The average person needs a little help with a set of reading glasses. However, for visually impaired people in this group, they will need additional eyeglass focusing power in their glasses. It is the additional eyeglass magnifying power and the closer working distance that project the larger image onto the retina.

The younger visually impaired still have the ability to focus up close, but wear reading glasses for their magnifying power. Although they can focus up close without visual aids, the focal distance of the magnifying glasses requires that any reading material needs to be held closer.

For people with poor visual acuity, the first adaption technique learned is to get closer to better see the details.

Eccentric Viewing

The macula is the central area of vision which has the ability to detect the detail needed for daily living tasks, especially reading. Eccentric viewing is an adaption technique of using another location in the retina as the area of fixation for visual tasks (also known as eccentric fixation). Typically, people who utilize this technique are those who have lost the use of their central vision area, which is the normal area of fixation.

Contemporary life is a printed society, starting with education and continues with work, communication, and activities of daily living. Learning eccentric viewing is a necessity, for those with impaired or central vision loss, and is the skill used during training regarding the use of magnifying devices. Adapting the technique of eccentric viewing can not only help with reading, but can also help with localization, mobility, and distance viewing, like watching television. It is a way for people with poor visual acuity to re-engage with their lives in order to maintain independence and prevent isolation.

Those who have lost their central vision are people who have macular degeneration, Stargardt's Disease, or Best's Disease. Other conditions which may affect the macula include diabetes, optic neuropathy, and optic neuritis. Someone with these conditions would be successful only if both maculae were affected. If one eye still has usable central vision, the natural reflex is to use the residual central vision of that eye. In that case, it would be frustrating to try to develop eccentric viewing. Another determining factor for success is the ability to locate a healthy retinal area to use for eccentric viewing. Someone that has large areas of vision loss, including the macula, may have more difficulty locating an area for eccentric fixation.

The peripheral retina, because of the type of photoreceptors and the way its neurons are wired, does not have the capability for fine visual discrimination of detail like the central vision area. The further away from the macular area, the less detail that can be identified. That means that someone with macular degeneration, but an otherwise healthy peripheral retina, may be only able to see 20/60 using eccentric fixation. It is precisely this reason why eccentric viewing must be combined with magnification.

Many who lose their central vision, especially those who lose it over a period of time, may naturally develop eccentric viewing. This is likely a survival mechanism. People who do not develop it independently, like those who had a sudden loss of vision, will need training. Initially this can be difficult. The natural tendency is to use the central vision area. This must be un-learned and a new area of fixation must be adapted. It is almost like you have to re-train your brain, and this takes time, practice, and patience. You will become aware of eye muscles you never knew you had before.

Training someone to adapt eccentric viewing is the domain of rehabilitation and occupational therapists. However, here is a little head start if you want to start your training.

The first step is to optimize your vision, that is, wear your best updated prescription reading glasses. Hold the following chart a distance of about 16 inches (40 cm). If your reading glasses' prescription is 'strong', you may need to hold the chart closer, which is the optimal focusing distance for your glasses. You should ensure that lighting is optimal and that the chart itself is well lit.

Nest, fix your central vision on the **+** sign. The plus sign may become blurry, distorted, or disappear altogether.

Now observe what you can see. Without moving your eyes, try to read one short word that is closest to the central area. If you can't read anything there, mentally observe a little further out and try to identify what you can see.. Can you identify any word? Do any of them seem to be easier to read than the others?

HIGH-LEFT HIGH HIGH-RITE

HIGH-LEFT HIGH HIGH-RITE

HIGH-LEFT HIGH HIGH-RITE

HIGH-LEFT HIGH HIGH-RITE

LEFT LEFT LEFT LEFT + RITE RITE RITE RITE

DOWN-LEFT DOWN DOWN-RITE

DOWN-LEFT DOWN DOWN-RITE

DOWN-LEFT DOWN DOWN-RITE

DOWN-LEFT DOWN DOWN-RITE

If you were able to pick out a word or two, make a mental note as to where it was located. Now try it again with the next chart. Remember, place your central vision area, again over the + sign, and observe what you can see.

NORTHWEST NORTH NORTHEAST

NORTHWEST NORTH NORTHEAST

NORTHWEST NORTH NORTHEAST

NORHTWEST NORTH NORTHEAST

WEST WEST WEST WEST + EAST EAST EAST EAST

SOUTHWEST SOUTH SOUTHEAST

SOUTHWEST SOUTH SOUTHEAST

SOUTHWEST SOUTH SOUTHEAST

SOUTHWEST SOUTH SOUTHEAST

Did you find a word or two in the same area as the first chart? If yes, congratulations you have found a possible Preferred Retinal Locus (PRL), in other words, an area you can train yourself to use for eccentric viewing.

Now, let's try the technique in reverse. Keeping in mind which word and area you read, as you will be placing your central vision in the opposite direction. For example, if the word you read in the first chart was DOWN, and it was the second one below the + sign. So in this case you would be placing the central vision area 2 rows up which is the opposite direction (the bold **+** sign in the chart for emphasis), to view the word "look" by eccentric viewing.

+ + **+** + +

+ + + + +

+ + LOOK + +

+ + + + +

+ + + + +

Or if you saw the word HIGH-LEFT in the first chart, which was one up and to the left, you should look down one and to the right. In this case, you will look at the **+** sign one down to right to observe the word "Look".

+ + + + +

+ + + + +

+ + LOOK + +

+ + + **+** +

+ + + + +

Now try it with the next chart.

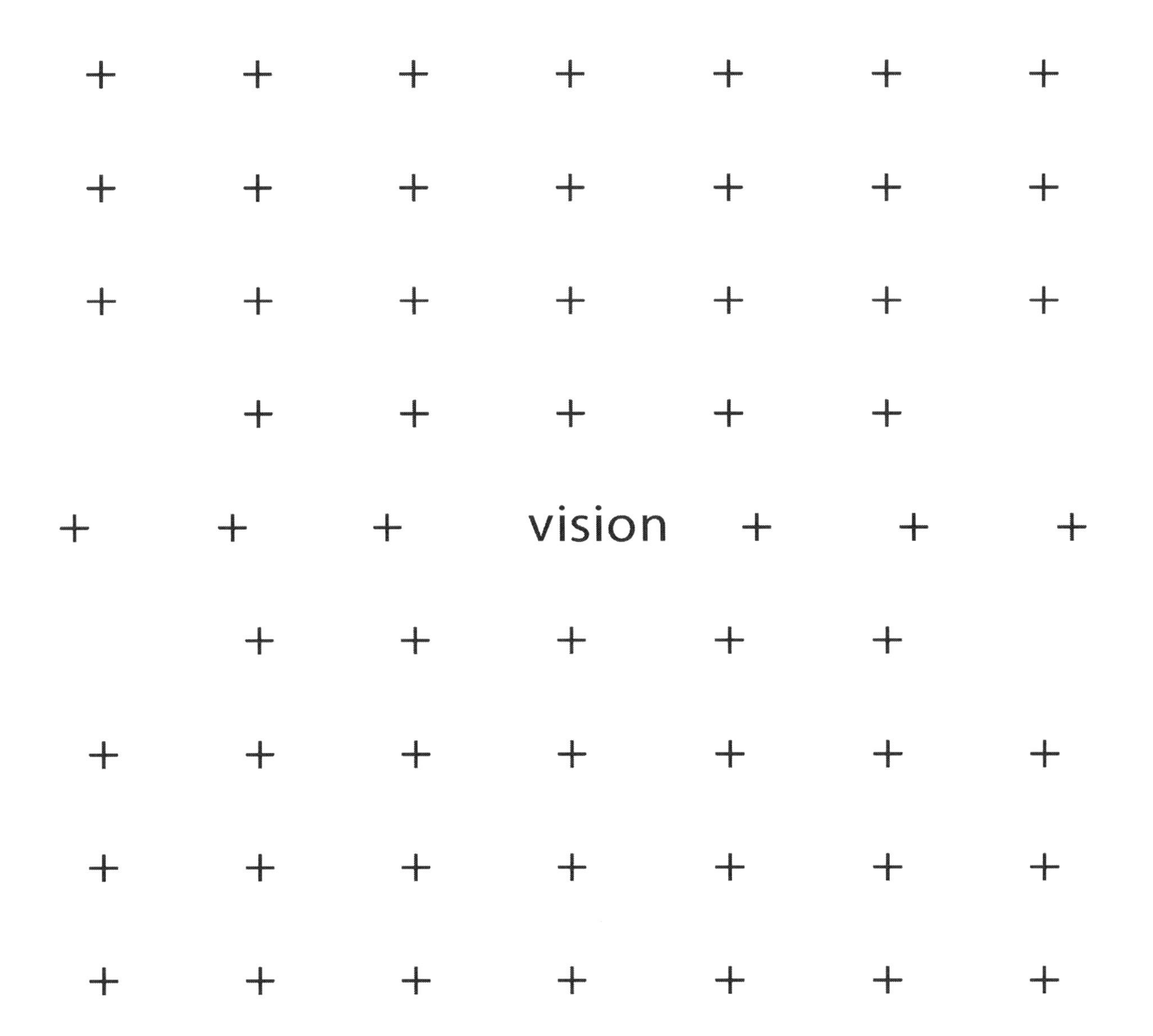

If you were able to move your impaired central vision to one of the other **+** signs, and see the central word, you used eccentric viewing.

The next phase is practice. It is best to hold your gaze steady, and move the grid, from right to left, as you would do to read normally. If moving the grid is too difficult or awkward, you should move your head. Remember to hold your gaze steady and try not to follow by moving your eyes.

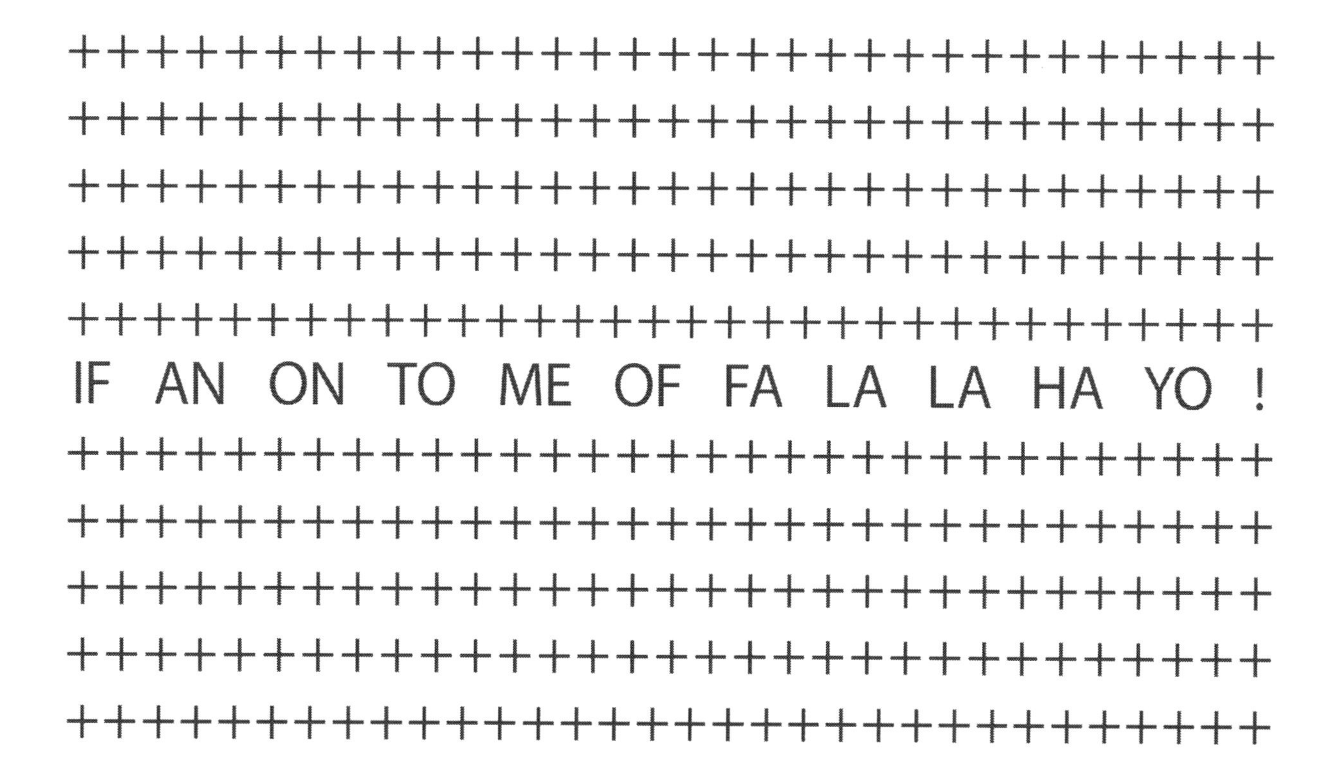

IF AN ON TO ME OF FA LA LA HA YO !

Learning this technique takes time and patience. Try it using a distance target, like a television. Using what you learned from the charts above, try it by placing the impaired central vision area on the corresponding section of the frame of the television. Now, as best you can, experiment by following the frame of the television. Your Preferred Retinal Locus, the PRL, should be the same as your reading PRL. Practice, because consistency is the key.

The goal of eccentric viewing is to enhance your reading abilities, and with practice, increase your reading speed. The greatest challenge of vision loss is not being able to read. It effects every aspect of our lives. Although getting closer and magnification are still necessary, eccentric viewing is a fundamental skill of adaption. Believe it or not, it can become second nature with practice.

Scanning

Scanning is a technique in which eye movement is used to compensate for the loss of the peripheral visual field, or used by those with poor visual acuity in order to gather information. Scanning can be defined as the organized, intentional pattern of eye movements, as opposed to a random hit or miss approach. People who use scanning are typically those with significant visual field loss, like those with retinitis pigmentosa, or hemianopsia.

Scanning is used to:

1. Localize where you are in an environment. Walk into a room, you would scan the area to determine if it were a small office or a large auditorium. By scanning, you can also determine where furniture, obstacles, and the exit doors are located.
2. Search for an object or person by scanning the environment. Contrast and lighting come into play when scanning a visually busy, or dynamic, moving environment.
3. Gather information by scanning, especially up close. This is helpful for gathering details of an object, image, reading material, or someone's face.

Scanning is done in an organized pattern of eye movements. Various patterns of horizontal and vertical scanning patterns are implemented. When scanning an environment, the eyes and/or head moves horizontally, say from left to right. Then the eyes drop stepwise, and a sweep of the scene is repeated. Once sufficient information is gathered horizontally, additional object information can be acquired by switching to a vertical scan of the area of interest. This full-field scanning technique works for people with contracted visual fields.

When searching for an object, you should first scan horizontally and then scan vertically. Say you know the clock is above the door, you should horizontally scan the room finding the door first, then scan upward. In this instance, tracing comes into play. Tracing is finding an edge of an object and then following the edge (or boundaries) to gather additional information. When walking on a sidewalk, the line of grass to the side is used as a guide for staying on the straight and narrow. Just like in a dark movie theater, you use the little lights on the edge of the aisle to guide you to your seat.

Someone with poor visual acuity or someone who uses eccentric viewing may scan an object up close to gather more detailed information about a face, a photo, a sign. or an object of interest with details. The scanning can be combined with tracing, by following lines or interesting details, to put together a complete mental picture.

Following a moving object with your eyes is called tracking. Tracking an object or a person for changes in their movement or direction can help with anticipation and an appropriate reaction. Tracking someone walking in front of you, or watching a car pass before you cross the street, helps us move safely in our environments.

For people with a large area of visual field loss, like a hemianopsia, they would develop a specialized scanning technique of looking rapidly to the area of field loss in order to compensate for the lack of vision in that area. These rapid, saccadic eye movements in the direction of the visual field defect, helps to keep you aware of surroundings and movement in that area of vision. The saccades (rapid eye movements) should be frequent, quick, and consistent and are similar to the eye movements of a driver using their side and rear view mirrors. The car's mirrors are used for the same reason; to help the driver visualize blind spots around the car.

Scanning affectively requires efficiency and smoothness like eccentric viewing, this training takes time, practice, and lots of patience. Scanning is a visual adaptive skill that can be utilized by someone who understands the extent and location of the patient's visual field loss. A rehabilitation or occupational therapist can recommend the best technique for compensating for visual field loss.

All Ears and Hands on Deck

Vision is just one of our five senses. Vision is a dominant sense, occupying a large part of the real estate of our brains. The other senses are hearing, touch, smell, and taste. While some activities involve just one sense, like reading, most activities of daily living involve multiple senses simultaneously. When we eat, we not only taste, but the smell adds to the enjoyment. When listening to music, we not only hear, but might sense the vibration from the sound. Input from multiple senses gives us a total picture of our surroundings or of an event.

Ever hear someone say that when you lose your vision, your hearing gets better? Actually, it becomes better in the sense that a skilled person with low vision will pay more attention to auditory clues. Location, distance, and movement can be sensed by paying attention to what we are hearing. You would not scan an entire room if you hear that what interests you is making noise in the corner.

Our tactile sense can give us information about objects without even looking at them. You can find your primary hand position on the computer keyboard by feeling for the nubs on the letter keys of F and J. Once you learn the controls on your assistive technologies, you can easily find them by touch. Commonly, even normally-sighted people don't need to look down to button their shirts or zip up their pants.

Conclusion

Adapting visual skills, practicing adaptive techniques, and using other sensory input is an individual matter. This ability is dependent on many disease-related factors, including age of onset, severity, pace of progression, and also the presence of other disabilities. A child will have greater flexibility than an adult, as someone with adult-onset vision loss has visual memory and experience. An individual who has a slow, progressive loss of vision has more years to develop their compensatory skills versus someone affected by sudden vision loss. Those with multiple disables, such as hearing loss or movement impairments, may have greater difficulty developing alternative adaptive techniques.

A skilled person with low vision can become adept at using adaptive techniques. It becomes a way of life.

Just remember **Time, Practice, and Patience**

Resources:

Corn, Anne L, Koenig, Alan J., Ed. Foundations of Low Vision: Clinical and Functional Perspectives. AFB Press, 2000.

Lueck, Amanda Hall, ED. Functional Vision A Practi'oners Guide to Evaluation and Intervention. AFB Press, 2004.

Scheiman, Mitchell. OD FCOVD FAAO, Scheiman, Maxine MEd OTR/L CLVT, Whitaker, Stephen G. PhD OTR/L CLVT, Low Vision Rehabilitation A Practical Guide for Occupational Therapists. SLACK Incorporated, 2007.

CHAPTER 13

Selection of Optical Visual Aids

The eye examination and low vision evaluation have led up to this point, in which the examiner puts it all together to find those visual aids that are for your lifestyle. It is art and science mixed with trial and try again. The low vision specialist has the numbers they need to put together an array of optical, electronic, and non-optical options. There are many considerations, including age, type and extent of vision loss, tasks of daily living, tools needed for employment or education, physical limitations, and other health issues. Your input is essential for finding the right combinations.

There are a myriad that are optical aids and new innovations available for patients. A specialist may have a particular set or brand of optical aids that they work with, because they have had success with them. The patient is given instruction and allowed to try out the various types. If the right combination of lens powers is found, but it is difficult to use, a training period will follow. An occupational therapist or rehabilitation therapist will work with you to establish new skills through practice and repetition using the new optical aids. Other skills training may include the adaption techniques of eccentric fixation and scanning discussed in Chapter 12.

Throughout the training sessions, adjustments in lens magnification and even types of aids may be made. What you need to bring is a willingness to do the work it takes to increase your visual function.

Remember, there is no longer one set of special glasses that will solve for the loss of visual acuity and function. The average person with low vision will need three to four visual aids. Each aid may have a different power and a different working distance which is needed to comfortably function at a specific task, as established during the low vision evaluation.

The use of non-optical aids should also be considered.. Non-optical aids are things like tints, filters, large print, typo scopes, and other aids designed for activities of daily living. These are discussed in other chapters.

Although there is an aid for almost any task, a few carefully chosen ones will suffice. The aids do not need to be sophisticated or expensive. Your input into the selection process is the key to success. The role of the low vision doctor is to make power determinations and help guide you through the selection process.

Introduction: Defining Diopters and Magnification

The unit used to identify the power of a lens is a diopter. This is indicated as the capital letter D after the number. For example; 3D is a lens with 3 diopters of power. The power of the lens is its capability to focus light. A 6D lens has a greater focusing ability than a 3D lens.

The mathematical definition of diopter (D), is that it is the reciprocal of the focal length. D= 1/f, where f is the focal length, and the 1 is 1 meter. The focal length is that distance that the user of the lens has to hold the reading material to get a clear image.

A low vision specialist will use the diopter unit to help determine the focal length. For example, a +2.5 D eyeglass lens means the wearer must hold reading material at 40 cm (about 16 inches):

2.5D = 1/f, calculated as 1 meter divided by 2.5 = .4 meter or 40 cm. (1 meter = 100 cm, .4 x 100 = 40cm)

Some more examples calculating focal length:

+ 2 D	1 M / 2 D	=	.5 M or 50 cm (about 20 Inches)
+ 3 D	1 M / 3 D	=	.33 M or 33cm (about 13 inches)
+ 6 D	1 M / 6 D	=	.16 M or 16 cm (about 6.5 inches)
+ 8 D	1 M / 8 D	=	.125M or 12.5 cm (about 5 inches)
+12 D	1 M / 12 D	=	.08 M or 8 cm (about 3 inches)

Note that the greater the dioptric power, the greater its ability to focus. This results in a shorter focal length. The stronger the lens, the closer things need to be held to be seen.

Magnification is a little more complicated, as there is more than one way to define and measure magnification. Whereas diopter refers to the power of the optical aid, magnification refers to the size of the retinal image, with indicate how large it appears to your eyes.

There are several types of magnification:

Relative size magnification increases an object's size. Large printed reading material is a form of relative size magnification.

Relative distance magnification is simply moving an object closer or moving yourself closer, such as sitting closer to the television. If you are sitting 8 feet away, then move 4 feet closer and you have given yourself 2X relative distance magnification. (Magnification = 8 divided by 4 = 2X)

Optical magnification is the ratio between the actual size of an object and the enlarged image size through the optical system projected onto the retina (light sensitive area in the back of the eye). Most familiar is the 'X' designation. For example: 8X refers to the magnified image as being 8 times larger than the actual object.

When attempting to calculate the magnification power, a lot of factors come into play, such as the dioptric power of one or more lenses and distances between lenses, objects, and the eye. Magnification is a much more complicated concept than lens diopter power. A simplification of optical magnification is to approximate + 4D for 1X magnification. For example, a +20D lens would give 5X magnification. (+20D divided by +4D = 5X.) This is a very loosey-goosy way of looking at magnification, without considering relative size and relative distance.

Spectacle Selection

The visual acuity and refraction portion of the eye examination is the basis for the initial eyeglass prescription. The prescription is incorporated into glasses as either a single vision prescription or as a bifocal. A bifocal is used when there is a different prescription for the distance and for near.

The factors that determine what type of glasses that will be selected are:

1. Prescription, as determined by the refraction;
2. Type of vision loss;
3. Age;
4. Tasks for which eyeglasses are needed; and
5. Personal preference.

The distance glasses are derived from the prescription that gave you the best distance vision. Making the glasses 'stronger' for distance viewing is not applicable here. You will see later in the chapter, that improving vision for the distance is accomplished using binoculars, telescopes, or bioptics.

A chief concern for those who visit the low vision doctor's office is the need to read small or 'normal' size print. A young person, who still has the ability to focus up close, will learn to pull the reading material closer to enlarge the print by relative distance (the closer, the bigger the retinal image). If this reading distance does not give sufficient enlargement, glasses for magnification will be prescribed.

Those over the age of 43, who have lost their ability to focus up close, by virtue of age, will require a bifocal. Loss of vision may require magnification over and above the regular reading prescription that those with 'normal' vision require. Fair warning: as the power of magnification increases, the distance with which you will need to hold the reading material will decrease. That is, the stronger the lens power, the closer that reading material must be held. (Refer to the earlier discussion and table which shows the higher the dioptric power (D), the shorter the focal distance.)

For example, a patient with a regular reading prescription (or a young person with their regular distance eyeglasses) holds the reading chart at the test distance of 16 inches (40 cm) to read 'regular' size print. The low vision person, who has lost some visual acuity, can only read 20/125 (2.5 M) at that same 16 inches. This print is about the size of the larger subtitle print you might see in a magazine. The person wants to be able to read the 'regular' size print in the magazine and this is the goal. The low vision doctor calculates the near power to be +6.25 D to read that print size. This stronger lens power has the effect of increasing the size of the print so it can now be read. The consequence is that the +6.25 add has a focal length of 7 inches (18 cm) and must be held at that distance in order to see print clearly. Upon demonstration and trial, the low vision person will determine if this closer reading distance is something to which they can adapt, and if this close working distance is sustainable.

Why Prisms are Prescribed for High Power Spectacles

Reading at a close distance requires that the eyes are brought closer together, or converge in order to maintain a single image. High-powered near reading prescriptions can put a strain on the convergence system, leading to eyestrain and fatigue. Base-in prisms are prescribed and ground into the lenses to reduce the need for the increased eye convergence for the closer viewing distance.

The Advantages of incorporating the magnification into the eyeglass spectacles are:

1. Hands free (especially good for patients with tremors);
2. Easily portable;
3. Less conspicuous in public, except for the closer reading; distance;
4. Most people have a familiarity with eyeglasses; and
5. Comparatively larger field of view (compared to hand-held magnifiers).

The Disadvantages of high power reading glasses are:

1. Close reading distance;
2. May be heavier, because they are thicker, and may require the addition of prisms;
3. Difficult to walk wearing glasses with a high-powered bifocal segment, because of the blur in the lower half of the eyeglass; and
4. Powers higher than +6D cannot be made in a bifocal format, but must be done as single vision (near, only).

Frame Selection

There are generally two types of frames for reading glasses. The first is the full frame, which gives a wider field of view. This frame can be heavier because of the larger lens size, and must be taken off to see anything beyond the reading material. The half-eye frame, better known as "granny glasses," will be less weight. Because of their low profile in front of the eyes, the distance can be seen by looking over the eyeglass frame.

Those persons with field constrictions should have two pairs of glasses, one for the distance and one for near. The bifocal set into the lower half of the lenses has the effect of detracting from the lower field of view. Individuals with field constriction have concerns of mobility. They are best served by having distance glasses that are full field with no bifocal segment to make walking more challenging.

When Monocular Spectacles are Prescribed

Eyeglasses may be prescribed to correct just one eye (monocular vision). Binocular corrections are prescribed up to +12D. Monocular low vision spectacles are done for those who have vision poorer than 20/200 in the better eye, and require a magnifying prescription above +12D. Glasses with higher magnifications are done as monocular prescriptions. This is because using both eyes (binocular vision) with these lenses; it is not possible to fuse the greatly enlarged images when held so close to the eye, to form a single image. Monocular vision glasses avoid the discomfort of double vision. A balance lens will be placed into the eyeglass frame for the uncorrected, poorer seeing eye. It maybe frosted to suppress the vision in that eye.

Aspheric Lenses

A term that comes up frequently when evaluating the quality of lenses is the tern 'aspheric.' Aspheric lenses are usually found in higher powered magnifiers and spectacles. The higher the power, the thicker and heavier the lens becomes. These thicker lenses also have a smaller clear central zone, because of their very curved surface. Aspheric lenses are a special design, that is ground to maximize the central clear area, and to decrease the central thickness and weight. These lenses are considered to be a better designed high power optical lens.

Microscope Lenses

The type of lens used for high magnification is called a microscope lens, and is set usually (but not always) as a monocular prescription into a frame as spectacles. The term is misleading, but is used because the construction is of two aspheric lenses placed together. This is not apparent when looking at the lenses, but it makes for a thick lens, as the power of microscope lenses can go up to 80D!

<u>The Advantages</u> of the Monocular Prescription are:

1. Hands free;
2. Portable;
3. Maximizes the vision of the better eye; and
4. Best option for the highest spectacle magnification.

The Disadvantages of the Monocular Prescription are:

1. Very close working distance with high magnification;
2. Small depth of focus, meaning there is very little leeway at the focal point to adjust for head, neck, and shoulder positioning because of the high magnification; and
3. Reduced reading time

Photo:

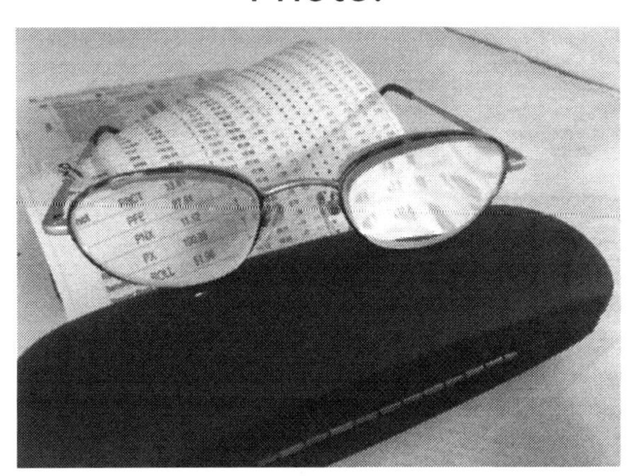

Microscope, high power lenses.

Add-On Specialty Lenses for Eyeglasses

Loupes-Monocular

Reading loupes can be used as a form of bifocal. They are high powered lenses that are small and attached to the eyeglasses, either on the frame or clipped over the lenses. Loupes can be either monocular, like the familiar jewelers' loupe, or binocular like those used by surgeons. Powers run in the +2.5D to +28D range (magnification of 1.7X to 7X). The loupe has the advantage of having the ability to be moved out of the line of sight when not needed for reading. They are also an inexpensive alternative. The down side is these small high powered lenses have a small field of view.

Clip-on Magnifiers- Binocular

These lenses are clipped to the frame and are suspended out in front of the regular prescription eyeglasses. Powers run from +1D to +4D. The reading distance depends on the combination of your prescription eyewear and the clip-on lenses. They have the advantage of being an inexpensive, do-it- yourself reading magnification system for hands-free reading. Similar to monocular loupes, they can be flipped up out of the way when not in use. The disadvantage is that they fit on some frames better than others. A small, light frame is less suitable than a larger, sturdier frame. Always be careful not to let the clip scratch the lenses. (It usually has a protective coating on the 'feet' of the clip.) These are an off-the-shelf devices, therefore they are not customized, and misalignment of the lenses-to-eye may result in some visual discomfort.

Photos:

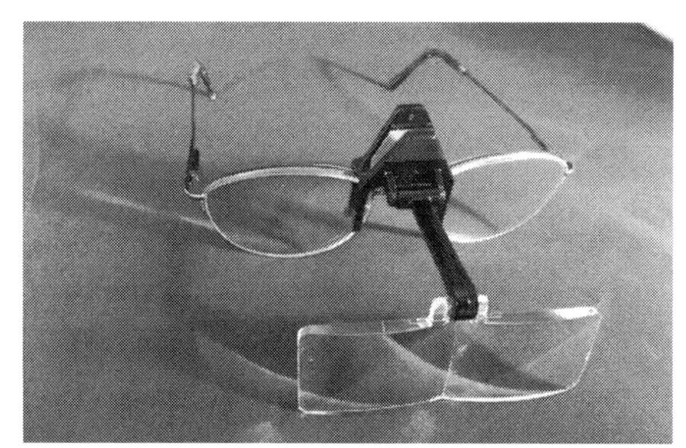

Clip on binocular loupes

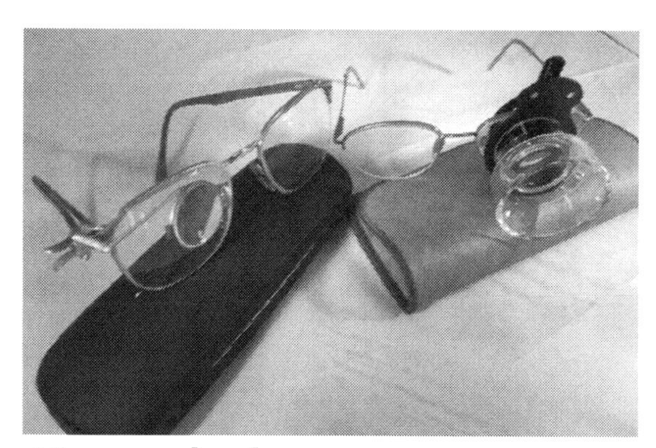

Monocular loupes

How to Use Magnifying Spectacles

First, the reading material to be viewed is held at a normal reading distance. Then it is brought toward the eye until the words are clear. This is the focal point of the lens. Instead of the usual head and/or eye movement, it is the reading material that is moved from right to left, then back to the beginning of the line by moving the reading material to the right. This technique of moving the reading material helps to keep the eye aligned in the center of the lens where the optimal lens power is located. The reading material should be well illuminated, with the light source located up behind the shoulder.

It is conceivable to end up with more than one set of glasses. If a prescription for bifocals is needed with a high add for near and the close working distance is not satisfactory, a lower power reading prescription (or just the distance prescription) can be used in conjunction with another form of magnification.

Introduction to Hand-Held and Stand Magnifiers

This section is a discussion of what we traditionally think of as magnifiers. These magnifying aids use lenses for magnification. Video magnifiers and electronic magnification are discussed in the chapter on electronic technology.

Hand-Held Magnifiers

These are probably the most frequently self-prescribed optical aids. The convex magnifying lenses are mounted in a plastic or metal frame. Some will have an attached handle. The types and models are numerous. Hand-held magnifiers can be small enough to fit into a pocket, hang on a chain, or even large enough to be carried around in a holster. They vary in shape, size, weight, and magnifying power. Some have built in illumination. It is recommended to use hand-held magnifiers with your distance eyeglass prescription (if you need distance correction). When bifocals or other reading prescriptions are worn, it changes the distance between the eyeglasses to the magnifier needed to get the clear image and therefore, the amount of magnification.

The trade off of using a hand-held magnifier versus a high powered spectacle is the field of view. Eyeglasses for magnification have a larger field of view. The size of the field of view of a hand-held magnifier is dependent upon the size of the lens. The size of the lens is dependent on the power of that lens. The higher the power, the smaller the lens becomes. The reason the lens gets smaller with increasing power is because of the weight. As a lens increases in power, it becomes thicker and therefore heavier. The smaller diameter of the high powered lens is to keep the magnifier from becoming weighty and uncomfortable to use

Hand held magnifiers come in powers of +3D to +80 D. The optimal magnification, in which the print is the clearest, is determined by the power of the lenses. This point is the focal length of the lens. However there is some variability in magnification, depending on:

1. How far the magnifier is held above the reading material;

2. How far your eye is from the magnifier; and

3. Whether you have eyeglasses on. Looking through your distance eyeglasses versus your reading glasses will give a different magnification.

The bottom line is that how you use a hand-held magnifier determines the amount of magnification. I told you that magnification can get complicated!

Fresnel Prism Magnifiers

Fresnel prism magnifiers are whole page magnifiers, or the small 'credit card' size pocket magnifiers. Fresnel lenses are usually a plastic sheet with circular ridges. These wedge-shaped ridges are prisms that redirect light and images. (The lenses of a lighthouse are a giant Fresnel lens that magnifies the light.) Magnifiers comprised of Fresnel lenses are good for being compact, light weight, and generally inexpensive. Their drawback is they only come in low magnification, and the optical quality is not as good as standard magnifying lenses.

The Advantages of Hand-Held Magnifiers are:

1. Reading material can be held further away from the eye, versus the eyeglasses of equal power, where reading material must be held closer;

2. Convenient and portable, for use on an as-needed basis for extra magnification (things like shopping and menus);

3. Can be inexpensive and available from many sources; and
4. Can be used with or without reading glasses.

The Disadvantages of Hand-Held Magnifiers are:

1. Small field of view versus the magnifying eyeglass;
2. Not hands free;
3. Long-term reading can be more difficult, which requires more endurance. This is because of the hand and arm position required to hold the lens at the optimal magnifying distance from the reading material; and
4. Cannot be used by patients with tremors.

Learning to Use a Hand-Held Magnifier

Start with the magnifier placed on, or at least very close, to the page. Using the handle, draw the magnifier up, watching the image. The point at which the reading material appears the clearest with maximum magnification is the focal length of that lens. Moving the magnifier across the page, maintain a constant hand-with-magnifier-to-print distance. An arm rest, like the arm of a chair for hand and shoulder comfort, is helpful. If there is a shadow cast on the page, readjust the lighting such that the page is better lit from the side without the interference of the magnifier's shadow.

A quick tip to increase the field of view with your magnifier is to bring your eye closer to the lens.

As indicated before, some endurance is required to read long term with a hand-held magnifier. This is the first type of magnifier people try because they can be inexpensive and are sold in many places. Often the quality of these magnifiers is poor. These inexpensive hand-held lens may not be optical grade, meaning the lens may have distortions, aberrations, and very small areas in which the focus is actually clear. This is often the case with the magnifying eyeglasses found in department stores. It is for the above-referred reasons that many people give up reading, with claims that "magnifiers don't work. "

Photos: There are many other options,

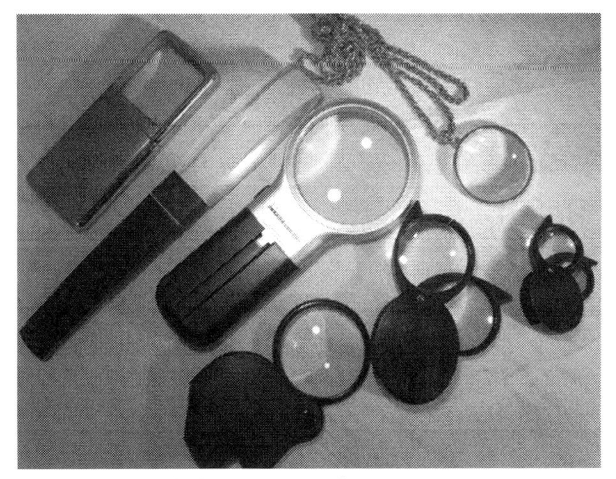

Hand held magnifiers

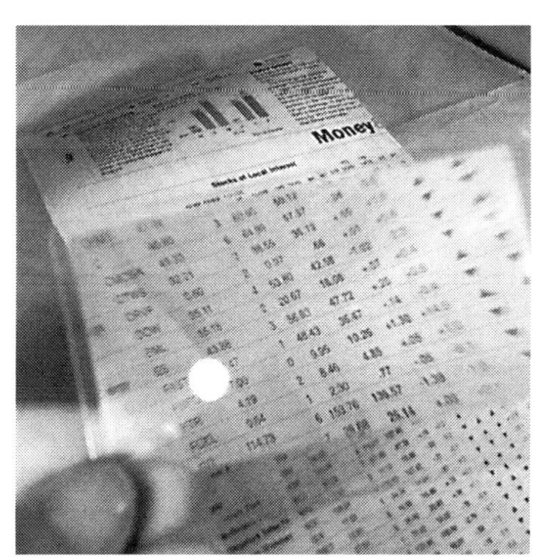

Credit card size Fresnel

Stand Magnifiers

Stand magnifiers utilize lenses like the hand- held magnifiers, but instead of a handle, they are mounted on a support system. The height the lens is from the base is a pre-focused distance, unlike the hand-held magnifier, where the user can adjust the height of the magnifier to focus. This pre-focused distance allows the user to rest the stand magnifier on the reading material and slide it along the page.

The lens is mounted in a position that requires that you must look down on it. For long-term reading, this could be an uncomfortable head and neck position. It is recommended that the user places the stand magnifier on a tilted surface, like a clipboard, tilted desk top, or lap desk.

Those people that require a reading prescription will need to use it with a stand magnifier. The focus of the magnifier is dependent on the eye-to-lens distance, and must be maintained in order to keep the reading material clear. When selecting a stand magnifier, your low vision specialist will help match the reading add of your eyeglasses to the magnifier for optimal working distance and field of view.

There are many types of stand magnifiers. Most of these are best left at home, as they are far too cumbersome to carry around. They can be inexpensive or surprisingly expensive. They can be non-illuminated or illuminated. The support stand of the magnifier when used, can throw a shadow on the page. Users who are bothered by this decrease in light or need higher contrast, will find the illuminated stand magnifier helpful.

The illuminated stand magnifiers can utilize incandescent, halogen, xenon, or LED lights. These light sources differ by color temperature. Incandescent, xenon, and halogen lights are warmer, more yellow hues, while LED lights are more white light. Halogen is the brightest, and consumes the most energy, and most likely will need to be plugged into electrical current (AC). LED requires less energy, can run on batteries, and LED bulbs last longer. For these reasons, LED illuminated magnifiers have become the most popular.

There are specialty stand magnifiers. The bright-field is a domed lens that looks like a paper weigh. It has the ability to gather the light to brighten the field of view. This is a lens favored for use by children. The dome power is usually in magnifications of 1.8X and 4X, in glass or acrylic.

Bar magnifiers are half-domed bars good for use on bottles, syringes, and are portable for menu reading. These are best for those with only a mild vision loss and/or constricted visual field, as the magnification is low. These magnifiers have low magnifying powers of 1.8X and 2X. Interestingly, they magnify greater in the vertical direction than horizontal.

<u>The Advantages</u> of the Stand Magnifier are:

1. Fixed focus, allowing it to rest on the page;
2. Used with a standard reading prescription;
3. Better for those with physical limitations (unsteady hands);
4. Good option for young children ; and
5. Many types to choose from.

<u>The Disadvantages</u> of the Stand Magnifier are:

1. Reduced field of view (versus magnifying eyeglasses);

2. May require an awkward head and neck position to look down on lens unless the user has a tilted work surface;
3. Less portable, especially if it needs to be plugged in for illumination;
4. Supporting stand can block light if not properly illuminated; and
5. People require a reading prescription. Adequate magnification is dependent on coupling the reading prescription with the correct stand magnifier.

Using the Stand Magnifier

The magnifier is simply placed over the top of the reading material on a flat surface, and slid across the page. Those requiring a reading prescription will need to wear their lenses. The user must keep a fairly constant eye–to-lens distance to keep the reading material clear. Moving the eye closer to the lens only increases the field of view minimally, and may cause the image to blur. This type of optical aid is best suited for short-term use like scanning. Stand magnifiers might be used to scan the phone book, recipes, newspapers, and the mail.

A quick tip: if you find yourself lifting the magnifier off the page, you need a stronger stand magnifier lens.

Thus far, the most common types of optical reading magnification have been discussed. There are other options for long-term reading. These are things like reading telescopes, CCTVs, video magnifiers, and computer-aided reading programs. Reading telescopes will be covered in the next section. The other reading options will be covered in the chapter on electronic technologies.

Photos:

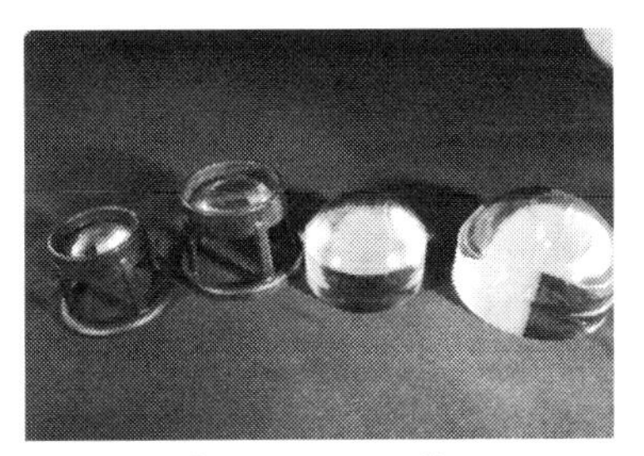
Stand magnifiers

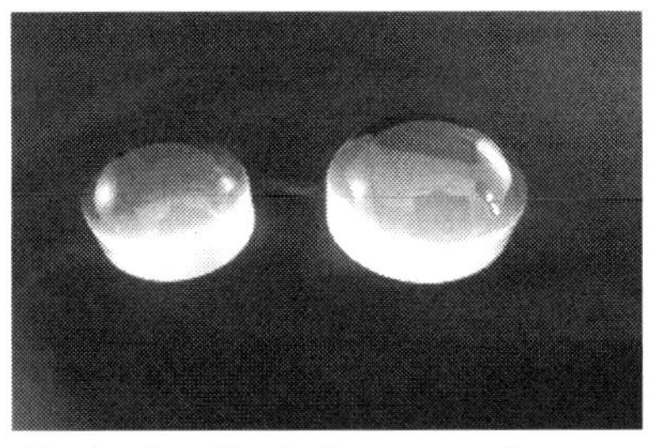
Brightfield stand magnifiers

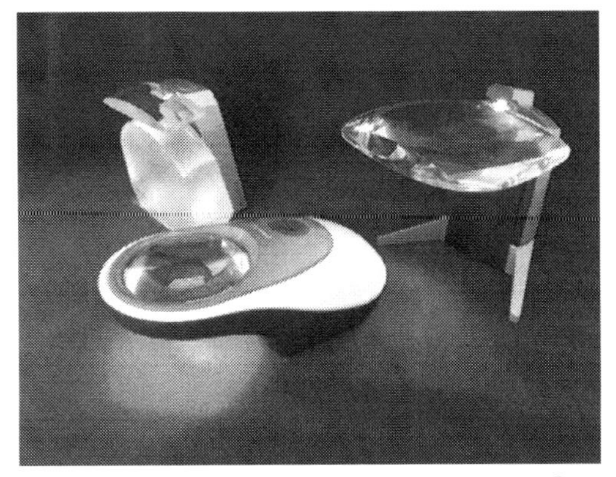
Illuminated stand magnifiers

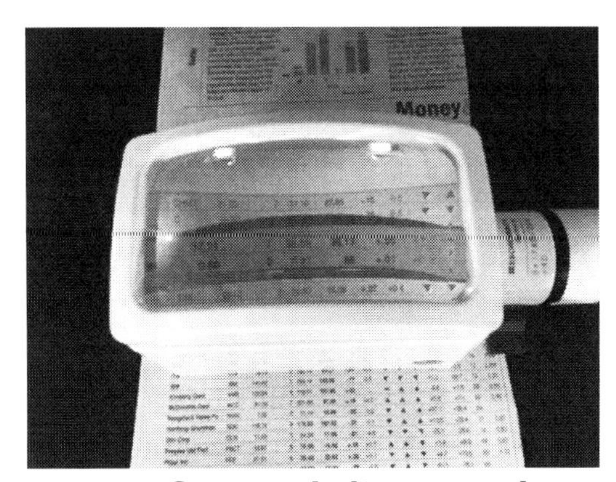

Magnifier with line marker

Telescopes

Telescopes are optical aids designed to improve distance viewing, or can be adapted for intermediate or near reading. While there are many options for near viewing, there are only a few multi-lens systems designed for far and intermediate distance magnification. These systems include telescopes, binoculars, and bioptic telescopes.

Telescope is a term used to describe a lens system that utilizes two lenses, typically an objective lens and an ocular lens. Telescopes are generally used for distances of 10 feet or greater. The field of view is small, almost like looking through a keyhole. They improve far vision by enlarging the distance objects and bringing them closer. The selection of a telescope is determined by the low vision specialist and you, based on your visual acuity and for what activity the telescope is needed.

What you need to understand about telescopes is that the stronger the telescope power, the smaller the field of view. Also, the thicker stronger lenses will transmit less light to the eye, making the distance details dimmer. This can be difficult for those with decreased contrast sensitivity. This is an optical aid where stronger is not necessarily better. The specialist will match your requirements with the minimum power needed to helps you, and that gives the biggest field of view.

Telescopes are generally not used when walking around. Not only because of their small field of view and the loss of side vision, but there is motion parallax, meaning a small movement of the head results in a seemingly large sweeping movement of objects seen through the telescope. These visual aids are primarily used in a stationary position for spotting or scanning.

Telescopes as Field Expanders

Those with field constrictions, such as retinitis pigmentosea and glaucoma, can use telescopes as field expanders. This is done by turning the telescope around and looking through the other end, which is normally the objective end. Looking through the objective lens has the opposite effect from looking through the ocular lens. It makes the field of view larger, things look farther away, and objects appear smaller. The drawback is that you must have fairly good visual acuity to see the miniaturized details in the distance.

Types of Telescopes

Within the category of telescopes there are those that are focusable or non-focusable, monocular or binocular, and hand-held or spectacle mounted. There are telescopes that can also be used for intermediate or up close viewing, either by focusing or by adding reading caps of various powers.

The general categories of telescopes are:

- Hand-held
- Clip on
    - Central
    - Bioptic
- Spectacle telescopes (Mounted Through the Lens)
  Full diameters
  Miniaturized (small telescopes)
    - Bioptic
    - Reading telemicroscopes
- Binoculars

Hand-Held Telescopes

These are the simplest form of telescopes. They are quite portable, and are valuable in aiding mobility. Some will even have a cord to attach to the neck, wrist, or a finger ring. The more frequently used power range is from 2x to 8x, but there are some hand-held telescopes with up to 20X magnification (which has a very tiny field of view of 3 degrees.)

It follows suit that the lower the magnification; the smaller and lighter the telescope. The more powerful the telescope; the longer and heavier it becomes, with a smaller field of view. Hand-held telescopes are for use on an as-needed basis for spotting distance objects. If you have a need for distance magnification, and are considering purchasing a telescope system, the hand-held telescope is a good starter lens.

The Advantages of Hand-Held Telescopes are:

1. Portable;
2. Good aid for spotting when on the move;
3. Can be inexpensive; and
4. Can be an effective training tool for learning to use a telescope.

The Disadvantages of Hand-Held Telescopes are:

1. Require at least one hand to hold steady;
2. Can be difficult to focus; and
3. Monocular (for use by one eye only).

Clip-On Telescopes

Clip-on telescopes are mounted on the front of your regular eyeglass distance prescription. They may look like a hand- held telescope, mounted either centrally or in what is generally called the bioptic position. Clip-ons are usually mounted on the glasses by a clip or ring that is fitted over and screwed in position to secure it to the eyeglass lens and frame. This option can be removed from the eyeglasses, but a screwdriver is required.

Centrally mounted clip-telescopes, referred to as sporting glasses, are an option for viewing when in a stationary position, but are not designed for walking around. Telescopes mounted just above the direct line of sight, are said to be in the bioptic position. The bioptic position is just above the pupil and is mounted with an upward tilted angle. This positioning allows the user to merely drop their chin closer to their chest and that way the telescope is moved into position to be seen through. The angle should be optimal for viewing straight ahead. While a centrally-located telescope is for constant use in a stationary position, a bioptic is used intermittently when walking or driving.

The bioptic used for driving is a monocular system, and is used for spotting signs and signals by the low vision driver. Bioptic telescopes can be binocular, but this is not the type permitted for driving. Bioptics are the only type that are designed for walking around, since lower and side (peripheral) vision is unimpeded.

There is a clip-on bioptic style telescope, designed by Ocutech, which is mounted on the nose bridge, and does not resemble a standard clip-on. It is a monocular lens that has the appearance of a horizontal bar mounted at the top of the eyeglasses. It is lightweight and less obtrusive than a comparably powered clip-on telescope. Bioptics will be discussed again under low vision driving.

The Advantages of Clip-on Telescopes are:

1. Hands free
2. Prices ranges from inexpensive to expensive; and
3. Can be focusable.

The Disadvantages of the Clip-on Telescope are:

1. Only the lower powers of magnification (2X to 4X, and an occasional 6x);
2. Some models can be heavy and uncomfortable with long-term use; and
3. Ocular portion of the telescope is further from the eye, resulting in a smaller field of view.

Photo:

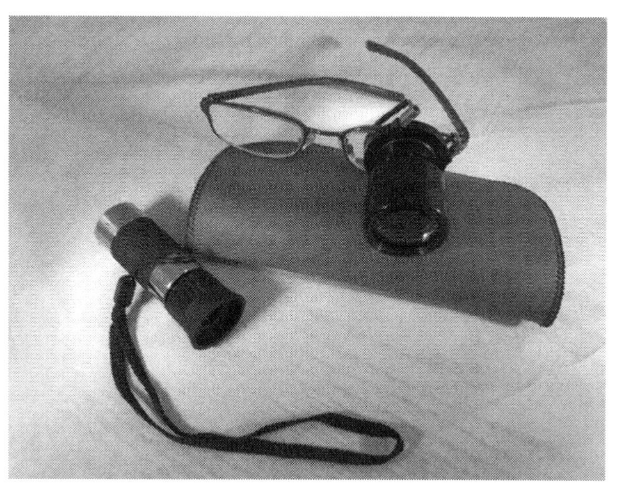

Hand held and clip-on monocular telescopes.

Spectacle Telescopes

Spectacle telescopes are a lens system mounted through a carrier lens in a frame. The system can be monocular or binocular. All types are custom made and tend to be very expensive. The measurement and fitting is performed by a professional trained in dispensing these telescope systems. The alignment needs to be precise, especially if it is a binocular telescope system.

An artifact of lens mounting is the ring of the mounting becomes a 'blind 'spot'. There is a jump between what is seen inside the telescope to the area just outside.

1. Full Field Telescopes. This telescope is mounted in the center of the line of sight. They have the widest field of view, with the close proximity of the telescope ocular-to-eye distance. These telescopes are good for distance viewing while stationary, such as watching sporting events, theater, and in the classroom.

2. Minaturized Telescopes. These are smaller lenses systems that have no outer housing. Similar to the full diameter telescope, the lenses are also mounted through the eyeglass, and can be monocular or binocular. The edges of the lenses are tinted black or tan, which helps to reduce extraneous light. They are light and less obtrusive than the other types of telescopes.

Spectacle telescopes are also custom and expensive. The lenses are defined by where they are mounted. They can be centrally mounted, bioptic position mounted (just above the pupil), or in the reading position as a telemicroscope (just below the pupil, like a bifocal).

The Advantages of Spectacle Telescopes are:

1. Hands free;
2. Customizable to maximize vision and visual comfort;
3. Binocular or monocular; and
4. Can be focusable or a reading caps can be added to the objective end to turn distance telescopes into near vision aids.

The Disadvantages of Spectacle Telescopes are:

1. Expensive;
2. Ring scotoma, a 'blind' dark ring, where the lens is mounted; and
3. Not a do-it-yourself vision aid, must be measured and fit by a competent professional.

Telescopes for Intermediate and Near: Telemicroscopes

Telemicroscopes are telescopes which can be used for close viewing. These can have the same effective magnifying power as high power magnifying eyeglasses (the previously discussed, 'microscopes'), but allow for reading material to be held at a further distance. Keep in mind the field of view will be smaller than high powered spectacles. There are three options for a telescope for near viewing:

1. Distance Telescopes Reading Cap Add-On. Standard distance telescopes can become reading telescopes by adding a reading

cap. The cap is an add-on lens, which is fit over the objective end of the telescope. This cap is designed by the manufacturer for that particular telescope, and is usually offered in two or more power options. The reading cap will determine how far away the objects or reading material should be positioned. One choice may be for intermediate (24-26 inches or 60 -65 cm) arms length working distance and one for near(16-18 inches or 40-46 cm) 'normal' reading distance. Some manufacturers offer a range of caps with intermediate to near focal distances.

2. Focusable Telescopes. Many telescopes can be focused from far to intermediate distance, and even closer, so they can be used as a telemicroscope for reading.

3. Dedicated Telemicroscopes. These are designed specifically for the near reading distance.

The Advantages of Telemicroscopes vs High Power Reading Glasses:

1. Reading material can be held further away; and

2. Expands the usefulness of your telescope.

The Disadvantage of Telemicroscopes vs High Powered Reading Glasses

1. Smaller field of view;

2. More conspicuous; and

3. More expensive.

Spectacle Binoculars

Spectacle binoculars are a low vision aid and are not the field-type binoculars purchased at sporting goods stores. These are smaller head mounted versions, and as the name indicates, for binocular (two eyes) viewing of either distance or near. The better quality units are customized, but there are those that are not custom. These off-the-shelf units which need only an adjustment for interpupillary distance (distance between the two eyes). The appearance of the head mounted unit can be awkward looking.

It is worth mentioning an inexpensive specialty binocular option, called the MaxTV. It is a two lens system, which has a set of lenses close to the eyes, like conventional glasses, and a second set of lenses mounted on temple extensions with an air space in between. There is an ability to focus each lens independently, to compensate for your prescription. As the name implies, they are designed for watching television at distances of about 10 feet, with a magnification of 2.1X. This option does not work for everyone.

The Advantages of Low Vision Binoculars are:

1. Hands free;
2. Focusable;
3. Widest field of view because both eyes are used;
4. Choice of customized or not customized;
5. Can be inexpensive (non-custom type, off-the-shelf); and

6. Adequate for long term viewing in a stationary position.

The Disadvantages of Low Vision Binoculars are:

1. Not attractive;
2. May be heavy and uncomfortable on the face with long-term use;
3. Measurement and fitting for custom, are best done by a professional; and
4. Custom will be expensive

Photos:

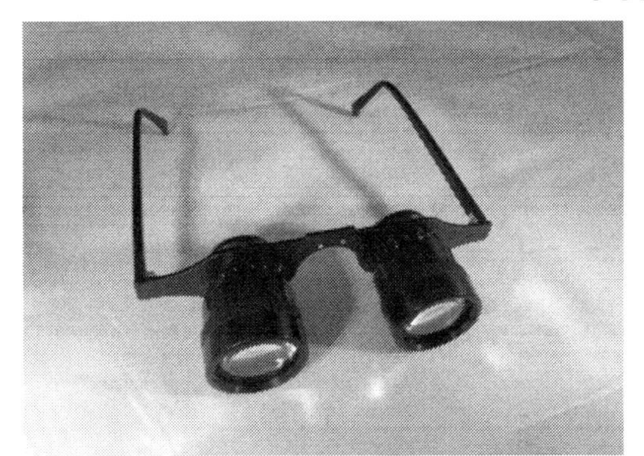

Spectacle binocular telescopes

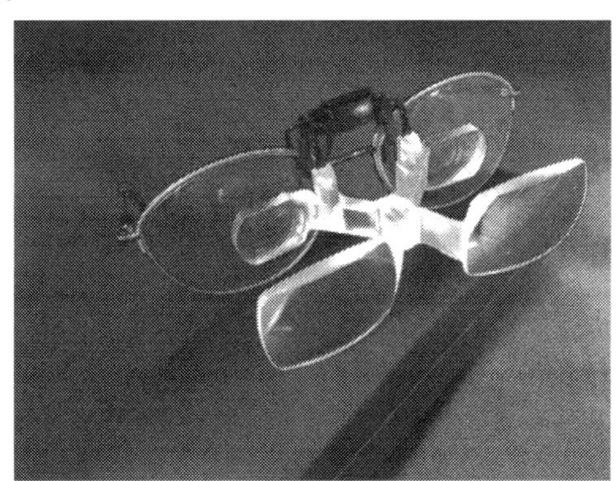

Clip-on telescope for near

How to Use Telescopes

First familiarize yourself with the telescope system. The correct end (the ocular end) to view through is the one that makes things look bigger and closer. Looking through the objective, makes things look smaller and further away. This technique of looking through the objective was mentioned previously as a way to expand the field of view for those who have visual field constrictions. The ocular end of a hand-held telescope may have a rubber eye cup. If it is a telescope with the capability to be focused, note where and how the adjustments are made.

First practice the eye-hand coordination. Start in a sitting position and select an object across the room. Keeping a steady gaze on the distance object, lift the telescope slowly into position in front of your better seeing eye. Your instinct will be to choose your dominant eye. If this turns out not to be your better seeing eye, you might be better served to learn to use the other eye. If you have an unsteady hand, pull your arm in close to your body, and rest the hand on your cheek. If it is a focusable telescope, bring your other hand up to adjust the clarity. Next, try the same exercise, standing up. Once you can do this proficiently in the close confines of the inside, you can move outdoors. Here you will learn the extent of your telescope's capability to focus on further objects. Locating an object in the distance, such as a sign, is called spotting. You can further your spotting skill by practicing viewing a stationary object, while in a moving vehicle. This is a skill that will be useful for bioptic driving.

There are a few other useful skills to develop when learning to use a telescope:

1. Tracing is following a line with the telescope, such as the edge of the curb, or the length of a pole.

2. Tracking is following a moving object with the telescope. Try following a meandering dog or bird in the yard (best not to track your neighbor around his or her yard, they may not understand you are 'practicing').

3. Scanning is assessing a larger object or scene by moving the telescope in a pattern, either horizontally (side to side) or vertically (up and down), to get a more complete view.

All three of these skills require that the eye, head, and shoulders move with the telescope as one unit so as to maintain the alignment of the eye to the object.

How to Use Telescopes for Reading

It would not be practical to use a hand-held telescope for reading. The reading telescope (which can be monocular or binocular) is head mounted, either on an eyeglass carrier lens or on its own frame mounting. The telescopes should be mounted in either a central straight ahead position or in the lower half of the carrier lens. The off-the-shelf type requires that adjustments be made to align the lenses to the eyes. There is an adjustment dial to align the telescopes in front of the pupil of each eye (interpupillary distance).

The telescopes will be either focusable to a close reading distance, or will utilize a reading cap. The distance that the reading material is to be held will be determined by the power of the reading cap. The low vision practitioner will help you find which reading cap is best for you.

The focusable telescopes are adjusted, first by choosing the reading distance, then focusing while keeping your eye on the letters. A binocular telescope system will require focusing one eye at a time. Do this by closing one eye and focusing, and then switching and focusing the other eye.

Reading telescopes require practice at finding the correct reading distance and moving the eye and head as a single unit. If more magnification is required, bring the reading material closer, and refocus the focusable type telescopes, or add a stronger reading cap for the non-focusable types.

Remember that good lighting is a standard requirement for low vision reading, as the multiple lens system of the telescope decreases the amount of light that reaches the eye.

Here are a Few Things to Remember about Telescopes:

1. The stronger the magnification factor, the smaller the field of view. The smaller the field of view, the more difficult the telescope will be to use for spotting. (For example, a 4X will be more difficult than a 3X, and telescope magnification above 4X can be very difficult to use.) Stronger is not necessarily better.

2. The dimmer the lighting, the more difficult a telescope is to use. It is easier to focus a brightly lit scene.

3. Holding the telescope close to the eye, maximizes the field of view.

4. The closer you are to the object of interest, the larger it will appear.

5. Develop a steady head, hand, and body positioning to minimize motion parallax. Motion parallax means a small motion of the telescope results in a large sweeping movement of the scene being viewed. This can result in visual motion discomfort.

6. Practice, practice, practice.

Fashion and Spectacle Telescopes, Bioptics, and Binoculars

The style can best be described as 'Retro.' Apparently the most durable and functional frames were designed in the 1970s. The fashionable color choices are things like 'gold,' chrome, and gunmetal. When I complained about style, I was told that the metal and plastic had to be a certain gauge thickness, with the lenses being a larger size. So if you are hoping for Gucci or Polo, stick to handbags and sportswear, because you are not going to find it at the low vision office.

Resources

Dickinson, Christine. Low Vision Principles and Practice. Oxford, Auckland, Boston, Johannesburg, Melbourne, New Delhi, Butterworth - Heinemann, 2002.

Faye, Eleanor E., M.D. Clinical Low Vision, 2nd Edition. Boston/Toronto, Little, Brown, and Company, 1984.

Faye, Eleanor E.,MD, Albert, Darren Lee, MD, Freed, Benjamin, OD, Seidman, Karen R., MPA, Fischer, Michael, OD. The Lighthouse Ophthalmology Resident Training Manual, A New Look at Vision Care. Lighthouse International, 2000.

Freeman, Paul B., Jose, Randall T., The Art and Practice of Low Vision, 2nd Edition. Boston, Oxford, Johannesburg, Melbourne, New Delhi, Singapore. Butterworth-Heinemann, 1997.

Nowakowski, Rodney W., Primary Low Vision Care. Norwalk Connecticut, Appleton & Lange, 1994.

CHAPTER 14

Light, Lenses, and the Eye

Light is the stimulus to the eye that produces the images that are perceived by the brain. Visible light is the optimal electromagnetic stimulus for the photoreceptors of the eye. We know there is a spectrum of electromagnetic radiation, which varies by wavelength. Visible light, which we would describe as 'white,' is actually composed of many wavelengths of electromagnetic energy. When each different wavelength of visible light is 'bent' at a slightly different angle, it results in a spectrum of colors we see as the rainbow. There is, however, other electromagnetic radiation that is not optimal for the photoreceptors of the eye to see. It is therefore, invisible to the eye. Those invisible wavelengths of light are the ultraviolet (UV) wavelengths, meaning 'beyond violet.' This is electromagnetic radiation beyond, but not seen at the violet end of the rainbow. The other end of the spectrum is the infrared electromagnetic radiation, which is also not visible to the naked eye.

Wavelengths of light are described in units of nanometers (nm = billionth of a meter). The visible light spectrum is between 750nm, which is the long wavelengths of red, to 400nm which is the shorter wavelength of violet. Ultraviolet radiation is an even shorter wavelength of 380nm to 250nm, and is higher in energy.

The 'near UV' area of the visible spectrum, 400 – 510nm, is seen as blue light. Recently this light has also come under scrutiny because it is at the end of the visible spectrum with the highest energy. The higher energy is what causes the problem for the eye. The normal eye, when subjected to intense or chronic UV radiation exposure can suffer photochemical changes to its tissues.(1) A diseased eye may be even more susceptible to UV and 'near UV damage.

We are all familiar with the labels on sunscreen products and sunglasses claiming UV, UVA, and UVB protection. The ultraviolet spectrum is divided into UVA (315-380nm), UVB (280-315nm), and UVC (200-280nm). UVC is the shortest wavelength and has the highest energy, and is absorbed by the ozone layer and the atmosphere. UVA and UVB pass through the atmosphere, even through a cloud cover, and can have a negative effect on our skin and eyes with intense or chronic exposure.

UV Light and the Eye

The cornea, which is the clear outer layer of the eye, is the first tissue affected by UV exposure. The high energy UV radiation can cause a very painful burn to the cornea. This can be experienced by a welder as a 'flash burn' from the high intensity, high energy welders arc. The sudden, intense UV light is absorbed by the cells of the cornea and can cause them to be damaged and die. A welder will tell you that it is very painful. Those who spend a lifetime working in the sun, especially those in a highly reflective environment (water, or snow), or live close to the equator, have chronic UV exposure which can result in degenerative diseases of the cornea and damage to the surrounding conjunctiva.

The next tissue to absorb UV light is the lens of the eye. Similar to the lens of a camera, the lens of the eye is a clear structure, located behind the pupil. Its role is to focus light to the retina in the back of the eye. Long-term exposure to UV radiation can change the structure of the proteins within the lens of the eye. (2, 3) This restructuring of the matrix of the lens results in a lens that is no longer clear. The cloudiness within the lenses is called a cataract. Keep in mind, UV exposure is not the only cause of cataracts.

UV light, which is not absorbed by the cornea or lenses, passes to the retina, which is the last structure to absorb the UV radiation. The energy of UV radiation, particularly the higher energy UVB, can damage the light sensitive photoreceptors and retinal pigment epithelium (RPE), resulting in a cascade of events leading to cell death. An inflammation of the retina (retinitis) can result from an intense exposure, like looking at an eclipse or a day spent looking at the highly reflective water or snow, which is the double whammy of direct sun UV radiation and reflected UV radiation. A lifetime of chronic UV and blue visible light exposure is thought to be one of the causes of age-related macular degeneration (ARMD). (4) Research suggests that not only is UV radiation harmful to the retina, but intense blue/violet radiation from the visible light spectrum may also be damaging to the retina.(5) This has become known as the 'blue light hazard.' (6)

The Blue Light Hazard

The "blue light hazard" refers to the accumulation of damage to the eye from the higher energy end of the visible light spectrum (High Energy Visible, HEV). The hazard is that while much of the UV radiation is absorbed by the cornea and lens, visible light in the blue/violet part of the visible spectrum makes it all the way to the very sensitive photoreceptors of the retina. These blue/violet wavelengths of the visible spectrum have higher energy than the green, which is termed medium energy, and red wavelengths, which are referred to as low energy. It is the higher energy of blue light (HEV) that is the 'hazard,' with the potential to cause damage to the light sensitive photoreceptors and eventual cell death with intense and/or long-term exposure. Exposure is constant and cumulative, that is to say, the negative effects may not be immediate, but accumulate over a lifetime.

Ocular Defenses

The eye has its natural defenses. The cornea and the lens of the eye absorb much of the UVA and UVB radiation which protects the very sensitive retina. Interestingly, as we age, our lenses take on a yellowish hue. This in and of itself provides additional protection for the retina, by blocking UV and some blue light. Those that have the most crystal clear lenses, like children and those who have had cataract surgery, have less of this natural defense, and in turn should be alert to eye protection.

The pupil is a diaphragm that opens or closes proportionally to the brightness of light. The pupillary reflex is to get smaller, admitting in less light to protect the retina.

The retina has the retinal pigment epithelium (RPE) and the macular pigments; lutein and zeaxanthin. The macular pigments filter out the UV and short wave blue light radiation before it reaches the photoreceptors. The RPE also scavenges for the potentially damaging free radicals.(7,8) These macular pigments naturally decrease with age. This is another reason why it is predominantly the senior population that develops age-related macular degeneration (AMD).

Anti-oxidants within the retina provide protection by sweeping up and neutralizing the reactive products, called free radicals of retinal metabolism. A diet poor in anti-oxidants, such as vitamin C and vitamin E, leaves the retinal tissues vulnerable to oxidative damage from high energy UV and blue light radiation.

There are risk factors that predispose someone to blue light damage, such as low macular pigment, tobacco usage, hereditary factors, and a lifetime of HEV radiation exposure. The diseased retina, depending on the disease process, may have these defenses compromised, resulting in a greater predisposition to damage by UV and blue/violet light.

Sources of UV Radiation and High Energy Blue Light

We are all familiar with the doctor's warnings regarding sunscreen protection for skin and sunglasses for protection against the harmful UVA and UVB radiation of sunlight. There are also indoor sources of UV and high energy visible (HEV) light radiation. Lighting choices have moved beyond the incandescent yellow-hued light bulb into various fluorescent and full-spectrum light sources, most notably LEDs (light-emitting diodes) and CFLs (compact fluorescent lights). The push has been, by government legislation, toward a move from the less efficient, less environmentally friendly incandescent light bulb to CFL and LED lighting, which use less energy and last longer. Unfortunately, both LEDs and CFLs emit a higher percentage of the HEV blue light. Whereas the old familiar incandescent light bulb emits 3% blue light, the CFL emits 25% and LED, 35%. Compare this to sunlight which is 25% to 30% blue light. (9)

The Importance of Blue Light

It is known that blue light does play an important positive role in our lives. It is not practical or possible to eliminate all high energy visible (HEV) blue light:

Blue light is responsible for our biological clock. The circadian rhythm, which is our sleep/wake cycle, has evolved from the appearance and disappearance of sunlight. Our pupils respond to a certain level of blue light. Hormones, melatonin, and mental status have all been tied to broad spectrum light exposure; which includes the HEV blue light.

Contemporary life has resulted in an increased level of blue light exposure through the use of technology. Our exposure to blue light has increased twofold; CFL bulbs are taking the place of traditional light bulbs in home and office, and LED lights are prevalent in cell phones, tablets, computer monitors, and television screens. Long-term use of these devices is responsible for the phenomenon referred to as computer vision syndrome (CVS) or digital eye strain (DES). These are characterized by eye strain, eye fatigue, headaches, and disruption of sleep cycles. Did you ever notice you have a hard time getting to sleep after staring at an LED screen before bedtime? It has to do with the afore mentioned blue light and the circadian rhythm. These devices have become, unavoidably, a part of our lives.

Those who are at risk for eye disease, or those whose ocular defenses are compromised by eye disease, need to be alert to the potential for damage due to UV and HEV blue light and to step up efforts to minimize their exposure.

Protecting Against UV Radiation and High Energy Visible Light.

UV Protection

Although we are naturally endowed with some ocular defenses to protect the retina from high energy radiation, it is not enough to totally defend against the sun's radiation, even on cloudy days. Many with eye disease are both light and glare sensitive, and are more comfortable with protective eyewear. Fortunately, it is socially fashionable and there are many choices available. How a lens performs is key, and if it happens to look good on you...Great!

There are three basic materials used for eyeglass lenses. They are plastic, polycarbonate, and glass. Plastic optical grade lenses for prescription eyewear are made out of a material called CR-39.

This type of lens, even in its clear form, offers some UV protection (wavelengths below 360 nm). Polycarbonate lenses are impact resistant lenses and often prescribed as safety eyewear for workers, children and monocular patients. They offer UV protection in its clear form (wavelengths below 380nm, and may be advertized as 100% UV protective). Both of these lenses block UV radiation by way of UV absorbers incorporated into the lens material. Glass lenses do not offer UV protection without the addition of a UV coating.

UV Coating

UV coatings are a clear, thin coat layer applied to the front and back of the lens to provide additional UV blocking capability, since plastic CR29 does not absorb all UV between 360 and 400nm and glass offers no UV protection. This is an option that is often bundled together with other lens options, like hard coats and anti-reflective coatings in what are considered premium lens.

Anti-Reflective Coating (AR Coat)

Did you ever notice that the people on television wearing eye glasses, even with studio lights overhead, don't have bright glare spots reflecting off their lenses like you did in the flash photo taken of you? That's because they have an anti-reflective coating on their lenses which makes the lenses nearly invisible. Not only does the AR coat give the eyeglasses a better look by reducing glare off the front of the lenses, but it also reduces the glare coming into the eye as well. An AR coating applied to the front of the lens will reduce visual glare giving better comfort and clarity. Likewise, an AR coat applied to the back surface of a lens (surface closest to the eye) reduces glare coming in from the sides that would otherwise be reflected into the eye from the back surface of the lens.

Individuals who wear polycarbonate lenses or those who opt for the lighter, thinner, hi-index lenses, may experience more internal reflections from within the lens material. An AR coat is also beneficial in helping reduce the glare associated with these specialty lenses.

Sunglasses

Here's what you need to know; not all sunglasses are created equal. Make sure if you are buying sunwear that is considered expensive; that the bulk of that expense should go to good quality UV blocking lenses and not just to the designer frame. A good quality, well-performing sunglass lens will block UV radiation, reduce glare, and give good contrast, resulting in not only protection, but comfort and clarity for the wearer.

Sunglasses should block 90% - 100% of ultraviolet radiation, and 75% - 90 %o of visible light.(10) Optical grade plastic and polycarbonate lenses, in their clear form, have UV absorbers integrated into the lens material. The darkness of the tint does not determine UV protection, but does determine how much visible light passes through to the eye. UV radiation is absorbed by other factors in these lenses that non-optical grade lenses may lack. If you do not get your sunwear from your eye care professional, and choose commercially-available sunglasses, make sure the lenses indicate UVA and UVB protection (ex.,UV 400) If you want to maximize what vision you have, be aware that non-optical grade lenses may have imperfections resulting in vision that is blurred or just not clear.

There are multiple considerations when choosing lens tints:

- <u>Darkness of the Tint</u>. The darker the tint, the less light is transmitted through the lens to the eye. If the tint is too light, you may find yourself still squinting in bright sunlight. A tint that is too dark may make visibility difficult in moderate sunlight levels. So consider your light sensitivity, and in what situations you will be using sunwear.
- <u>Color of the Tint</u>. Tints can change color perception.
- <u>Contrast Enhancement</u>. Compare a distance object to its background. The object should stand out from its background. Those with low vision should not expect their vision to be degraded if the tint is appropriate.
- <u>Glare Reduction</u>. Check for visible glare, either in the distance or off the lenses themselves. Glare reduces the comfort and clarity of vision. If you still feel the need to squint, consider some other glare reducing options like AR coats and polarized lenses.

Lens Tints

The two most popular and fashionable colors for tints are grey and brown. In the past green and vermillion, which is a rose colored lens, have also been popular. Every once in awhile you will see someone who prefers the yellow/amber color.

- Grey is considered to give the most normal color perception, and is best at reducing brightness. It does not increase contrast, and is best coupled with polarization for that reason. It is best used for moderate to brightly- lighted situations for distance viewing and for driving.
- Brown is also considered to give nearly normal color vision. It is better at blue- blocking, increasing contrast, and the distance still appears 'bright.'
- Green filters out most of the blue, and works well on bright hazy days. It has been popular for use in outdoor sports, due to the high contrast of red and yellows against green backgrounds (e.g., foliage, trees).
- Rose or Vermillion increases contrast and brightness. Darker tints are good for moderate to bright outdoor lighting. Light tints have been indicated for working under fluorescent lighting and computer screen viewing.
- Yellow lenses are total blue blockers, which decreases glare, and enhance contrast, but have the unfortunate effect of distorting all other colors. Yellow tints are best described as filters that are not used so much as sunwear, but are

best used when high contrast is helpful, like in the low light of morning or dusk. It is also useful as a tint for shooting sportsman, to cut the blue of the sky and increase the contrast of their targets.

- Amber/brown blocks blue light, gives good contrast, and in its darker tints can be used for moderate to bright sunlight. Because of the yellow tint, colors will be distorted. Be wary of driving with yellow and amber tinted lenses because of the distortion of the color of signal lights.

How the frame fits the face is important for protection against stray sunlight. The lenses should be large enough and fit close to the face, ideally a form fit that wraps around the eye area to decrease sunlight exposure from the edges of the lens and frame.

There is a whole category of sunglasses designed to fit over prescription eyewear. Several brands are composed of optical grade lenses for clarity with no lens induced distortion and offer 100% UV 400 protection and 100% polarization. They also have side shields along the temples, and the frame extends over and under the prescription eyewear to protect against stray light entering from the sides, top, and bottom. Although you may associate these large sunglasses with your grandmother after cataract surgery, the reality is that they are designed for anyone who wants maximum protection while still maintaining clarity of vision. The financial benefit is that they are moderately priced and since they fit over your eyeglass prescription, you do not need to invest in a dedicated set of prescription sunglasses.

Photosensitive Lenses

Photosensitive lenses have the ability to change from clear, or nearly clear, prescription eyewear to prescription sunwear. Specialized molecules embedded on the surface layer or within the matrix of the lens, are sensitive to UV radiation. These molecules react by changing configuration and in turn absorb light. The absorption of light changes the lens from clear to tinted. When the lens is no longer exposed to UV radiation, like going from outdoors to indoors, the molecules revert and the tint fades and the lens is once again clear. Even on a cloudy day, when you might otherwise not think sunglasses are necessary, they will react to UV that passes through the cloud cover. The advantage is that your prescription eye wear does double duty as a set of dress eyewear and sunglasses, giving you clarity, comfort, and protection, both inside and out.

The first photochromic lenses were made of glass, but photosensitive lenses can now be purchased in plastic, including hi-index and polycarbonate. The most well known is Transitions,® whose name has become synonymous with plastic photosensitive lens. The predominate tints offered by manufacturers of photosensitive lenses are grey and brown. They are made as prescription eyewear in single vision, bifocal, trifocal, and progressive lenses.

There are photosensitive sunglasses which are tinted, but when exposed to UV, get even darker in response. These are variable tint sunglasses.

Corning Medical Optics makes a specialty line of glass photochromic sunglasses called CPF GlareControl® lenses in tints designed for those with eye conditions, who have difficulty adapting to different light levels. Examples are:

- Yellow that darkens to amber to reduce high energy blue light and glare;
- Orange/amber that darkens to brown to aid visual function and reduce glare; and
- Red/amber which darkens to brown for those who are the most light sensitive.(11)

A low vision specialist can best help with specialty tint lens selection.

A few things to keep in mind regarding photosensitive lenses:

1. Although they quickly darken outside, in a minute or two, they can take 5 or more minutes to clear again indoors.

2. They do not fully darken in the car. The roof over your head and the windshield do not allow for UV light to hit the lenses directly.

3. They are temperature sensitive, and interestingly, perform better in cold temperatures than hot temperatures.

4. The capability to darken and lighten fully, wanes over time. Manufacturers say you can expect them to perform optimally for about 3 years.

Polarization

The polarization feature is linked to tinted eyewear. In bright outdoor sunlight, although sunglasses decrease the amount of light that passes through the lens to the eye, there are still glare spots. Glare is light reflected at various angles that reduces contrast. The polarized lens blocks glare off of horizontal surfaces, such as water, snow cover, or the hood of a car. By blocking horizontally-reflected light a polarized lens can give clearer and sharper visibility. Fishermen demand polarized lenses in order to reduce the glare of the water's surface, allowing them to see down into the water. Drivers can see better without the veiling glare off the road, hood, and dashboard. I believe polarized sunglasses helps to prevent wrinkles, as it keeps you from squinting.

Polarization is almost a necessity with grey neutral lenses in order to increase contrast. Consider that not all polarized lenses are created equal. It is not a point advertised, even among the premium lens products, but there is 100% polarized, and then there are those that offer only partial polarization.

Tints/Filters for Improving Visual Function for the Visually Impaired

Those with visual disabilities often experience extreme light sensitivity, disabling glare, and loss of contrast sensitivity. NoIR Medical Technologies® has a broad palette of lens colors and tints that have been prescribed for decades for various eye conditions. Some of these specialty lens tints are filters for increasing contrast and some are darker tints used for light sensitivity, contrast, and glare control. Filter colors and sunglass tint recommendations by NoIR® (No InfraRed) vary by eye condition. Selection of the appropriate lens tint is best done with the help of a low vision specialist. There are over 50 different lens choices, and selection is based on the eye condition and personal needs, with a little personal preference thrown in.

Contact Lenses and UV Protection

There are only a few contact lens brands that offer UV-blocking. That can be related to the lack of demand by patients and their doctors for this added benefit to contact lens wear.

For contact lens to be labeled as Class 1 UV-blocking, it must block 99% of UVB and 90% of UVA. These are American National Standard Institute Z80.20 standards adopted by the FDA.(12) Currently, only one manufacturer produces Class 1 UV-blocking contact lenses (some Vistacon® Acuvue® brands). Class 2 UV-blocking contact lenses must block 95% of UVB and 70% of UVA. Again, currently there are only a few lens brands, that can make this Class 2 claim.(13)

The benefit of contact lenses as a UV filter is that it protects the eye from stray light radiation that would otherwise enter the eye from the sides of a pair of eyeglass lenses. The drawback is that although soft contact lenses completely cover the cornea of the eye, the other tissues, like the conjunctiva and delicate eye lids, are still exposed to UV radiation.

Wearing UV-blocking contact lenses does not preclude the use of sunglasses all together. If someone is wearing contacts anyway, why not have the added benefit of UV protection? Contact lenses should be viewed as another line of defense, but not a replacement for sunglasses.

Protection from 'The Blue Light Hazard,'

The danger of chronic and intense UV radiation exposure from sunlight has been known for decades, and has been addressed with UV-blocking eyeglass technologies, both old and new. The explosion of digital technology since the turn of the century has brought up a new concern, and that is the high energy visible (HEV) light in the blue/violet range of the visible spectrum (400nm to 500nm). Too much exposure to light in this range is called the 'blue light hazard.' Compact fluorescent lights (CFL) and light emitting-diodes (LED) digital screens are the culprits. The concern regarding blue light is two-fold:

1. Eye Health. The blue light hazard refers to concerns about the future eye health of those who will spend hours, days, weeks, into years with indoor high energy visible light. This exposure is chronic and cumulative. There is mounting evidence that exposure to blue/violet light can have a negative effect on the lens of the eye and the retina. Because of its energy, blue/violet light has the potential to cause permanent damage to these tissues. Those in the low vision community, whose ocular defenses may already be compromised and are struggling to preserve their residual vision, need to address this potential source for retinal damage.

2. Eye Strain. Eyestrain has become common place for those who spend hours a day on these electronic devices in rooms lit by CFLs. Digital Eye Strain (DES) has visually related symptoms such as achy eyes, redness, blur, dryness of the eyes, headaches, eye fatigue, and accompanying neck and backaches. HEV emitted from these devices has been implicated as one of the causes of DES and potentially disrupts our natural circadian rhythm. Those with visual impairments, who in the past have suffered from eyestrain secondary to high prescription eyewear and magnifying lenses, which have their own issues, now join the ranks of those suffering with DES through the use of LED screens of both computers and accessibility technology.

   Some of these problems associated with DES can be alleviated by taking the following steps:

   - Make sure the screen is in a comfortable position, which should be slightly below eye level. This will help with eye, back, and neck aches;
   - Adjust the font to a comfortable size to relieve straining;
   - Adjust the backlight level. Decrease the brightness of your LED screen,. (it saves the battery, too);
   - Take frequent visual breaks: The 20/20/20 philosophy is: look at a distance of 20 feet, for 20 seconds, every 20 minutes; and
   - Get the most appropriate eyeglass prescription for the

computer working distance, and add to that blue blocking technology.

Blue Blocking Technology

As previously mentioned, blue light in the visible spectrum is a necessary part of our lives. It is important not just for the visible color blue, but is important for biological, non-visible functions such as our circadian rhythm, pupil reflex, and psychosocial functioning. Seasonal Affective Disorder (SAD) is a psychological disorder associated with the winter months, in which there is an extended period of time without sunlight.

In 2012, an optical manufacturer by the name of Essilor International,® in conjunction with Paris Vision Institute, looked at the high energy, short wavelength blue light spectrum in small increments. That is, the wavelengths just above UV in the range of 380nm to 500nm. They looked at what wavelengths caused damage, and what blue wavelengths were useful for biological non-visual function (circadian rhythm, pupil reflex, etc). The question was: Could a lens be created that filtered out the 'bad' blue light, but transmitted the necessary beneficial blue light?

First they identified the 'bad' HEV in the 415-455nm range as 'phototoxic.' But there was a narrow band in the 465-495nm that allowed for normal biological response to blue light without the damaging effects of the higher energy blue light. Lenses have since been created that absorb UV and blue light above 455nm. These lenses are transparent; they do not distort color vision like sunglasses, although a slight tint nay be seen. The manufacturer is careful to point out that not all 'bad' blue light is absorbed, but is reduced (about 20%).(9) These lenses will serve those who spend time indoors under CFLs, and use cell phones, computer LED screens, and monitor LED screens.

The lens specifically mentioned in the report was the Essilor Crizal® Provencia No-Glare® lens. I hesitate to mention lens brand names; but I will mention a few at this writing to give readers an idea of what to ask for. Manufacturers are constantly adding new technology, modifying features, and discontinuing or changing the names of existing products. You should keep that in mind. Those with blue blocking technology are:

- Crizal®Prevencia No-Glare® (Essilor);
- BluTech® (Eye Solutions Technology);
- Recharge® (Hoya);
- SeeCoat Blue® (Nikon);
- iBluCoat® (VCD Labs);
- UVARity ® (Laramy K-Optical); and
- Retinal Bliss Tech DES Coating® (Quantum Innovations).

These manufacturers do not claim 100% blue-blocking. These clear, natural looking glasses can help relieve eyestrain caused by blue/violet light.

There are a few other things you can do to reduce HEV coming off of LED screens, as we know yellow/amber tints block blue light:

- Place a yellow filter between your eyes and the screen. This can come in the form of yellow/amber slip-over colored specs, like Cocoons,®r Fit Overs,® NoIR® lenses, or SolarSheilds.® These have the benefit of providing 100% UV and blue blocking, with increased contrast.
- Blue blocking filters can be purchased for your computer screen. Type "computer screen filters, blue light" into the search bar on the internet search engine. An anti-reflective screen covers can help reduce glare off the surface of the device. Glare can contribute to eyestrain.
- Another option is to change the polarity on your device. White or yellow print on a black screen is easier on the eyes, especially at night. The ability to change polarity is a universal feature of CCTVs and video magnifiers.
- There is an app for that on mobile devices. Type into the search bar 'blue light filter app' to find one for your operating system. These offer to dampen blue light or change the color temperature. There are also apps to control the brightness of the screen. These offer to automatically decrease screen brightness as the day passes to night, or allow you to control screen brightness below the default settings. Search 'screen brightness control app.'

Conclusion

The optimal eyeglass prescription is important for visual acuity, but eyewear can be more than just that. Lenses with UV coating, anti-reflective coating, and blue light blocking technology can protect you from damaging UV radiation and high energy visible light. Tints and polarization, along with anti-reflective coating, can help with visual function by reducing glare and increasing contrast. Maximize eye protection with premium eye lenses, and adequate lens size and frame coverage.

Protecting your eyes indoors from artificial light sources that emit HEV can not only protect the eyes from the potentially damaging effects of long-term exposure, but the eyes should feel more relaxed, less strained, and enable you to fall asleep easier at night.

References

1. Liu IY, White L, Lacroix AZ. The association of age- related macular degeneration and lens opacities in the aged. Am. J. Public Health. 79:765-769(1988).
2. Zigman, S. Light damage to the lens. In: Clinical Light Damage to the Eye (D. Miller, Ed.), Springer-Verlag, New York, 1987, pp.65-78.
3. Lerman, S., Megaw, J. M., and Moran, M. N. Further studies on the effects of UV radiation on the human lens. Ophthal. Res. 17: 354-361 (1985).
4. Taylor HR, West S, Munoz B, Rosenthal FS, Bresseler SB, Bresseler NM. The Long Term Effects of visible light on the Eye. Archives of Ophthalmol.1992;110:99-104.
5. Reme CE, Wentzel A. Grimm C, Iseti HP. Mechanisms of Blue Light Induced Retinal Degeneration and the Potential Relevance for Age Related macular Degeneration and Inherited Retinal Diseases. SLTBR Annual Meetings Abstracts 2003.

6. Young RW. Solar Radiation and age-related macular degeneration. Surv. Ophthmol. 32:252-260 (1988).

7. Yu J, Johnson EJ, Shang F, et al. Measurement of macular pigment optical density in a healthy Chinese population sample. Invest Ophthalmol Vis Sci. 2012;53(4):2106-11.

8. Whitehead AJ, Mares JA, Danis RP. Macular pigment: a review of current knowledge. Arch Ophthalmol. 2006;124(7):1038-45..

9. Smick K, Villette T, Boulton ME, Brainard GC, Jones W, karpecki P, Melton R, Thomas R, Sliney D, Shechtman D. Blue Light Hazard: New Knowledge, New Approaches to Maintaining Ocular Health. Report of a Roundtable. March 16, 2013 New York City, NY, USA. **www.crizalusa.com/.../Blue%20 Light%20Roundtable_White%20Paper.p**...

10. UV protection. Home >>Patients and Public >>Caring for Your Vision >>UV protection Retrieved from **aoa.org**

11. What are Corning CPF lenses. Retrieved from **www.cpfglarecontrol.com/CPF_Lenses.html**

12. UV Protection with Contact Lenses. Home > Patients & Public > Caring for YourVision > UV Protection > UV Protection with Contact Lenses. Retrieved from **www.aoa.org/**

13. Cohen et al. A Closer Look at UV -blocking Contact Lenses. Contact Lens Spectrum, Nov 1, 2007.

14. Smick K, Villette T, Boulton ME, Brainard GC, Jones W, karpecki P, Melton R, Thomas R, Sliney D, Shechtman D. Blue Light Hazard: New Knowledge, New Approaches to Maintaining Ocular Health. Report of a Roundtable. March 16, 2013 New York City, NY, USA. Retrieved from **www.crizalusa.com/.../Blue%20Light%20Roundtable_White%20Paper.p**

CHAPTER 15

Electronic Technology

"Where there is a will, there is a way."

The discussion thus far has centered on the optical technology of magnifiers and telescopes that have long been associated as being the adaption technologies for visually impaired. These forms of assistive technologies have been around, in different forms, ever since optical jewelry makers realized they could magnify the printed word. Now in their wake, contemporary designers of electronic technologies have recognized the need of those who can benefit from technology used to magnify or present in audio form, the printed word.

Not only has there arisen a vast array of electronic devices to assist the visually impaired (assistive technology), but technology that adapted computers and cell phones to make mainstream technology accessible (accessible technology). The advent of e-readers and electronic tablets are now blurring the lines between assistive technology and accessible technology.

During this general discussion of electronic technology, I will resist, with a few exceptions, naming names. Technology is on the move. Manufacturers are constantly adding new products, new features to established products, changing their names, and discontinuing products. An invaluable source to keep abreast of technology changes is *ACCESSWORLD,* which is an online journal which evaluates and reviews accessible and assistive technology. It is found on the American Foundation for the Blind website under the technology section.

Similar to optical magnification aids previously discussed, there are different categories of aids for different tasks. There is no one technology option that does it all. Here is what you will learn quickly, as you evaluate your electronic technology options; there is no inexpensive choice. You will need to weigh the cost vs. benefit for these more pricey aids. I will tell you having access to electronic devices has opened up the world. It is a must for students to keep up with classmates, and it can keep adults employed. Electronic devices can increase your reading time, reading speed, decrease visual discomfort, and overall grant you access to what everyone else takes for granted.

CCTV/Video Magnifiers

Closed circuit televisions (CCTV) have been around for several decades now. Along with the changes in technology, CCTVs have gotten better, offering more flexibility and options. There is an entire category ranging from the familiar desktop behemoth, to the small pocket size models, with several other options in between.

No matter what the size, CCTVs are basically a camera, a screen to view what the camera 'sees,' and a light source for the field that the camera views. The general categories to be discussed are:

1. Desktop CCTV;
2. Portable Table Top CCTV;
3. Computer/Laptop Compatibles CCTV; and
4. Hand-Held video Magnifiers.

1. Desktop CCTV

These are the best options for long-term reading. Most desktop models have a movable table, called an XY table, mounted under the camera and monitor. This XY table glides side to side (X direction) and forward and backward (Y direction). The user can sit back in the chair, adjust the magnification, and read by moving the text back and forth under the camera, and by virtue of the monitor, enjoy a large field of view. Being able to see more words at a time can increase your reading speed. The table can also be locked in position, and used for other activities such as writing and hobbies. Similar to the personal computer, this model requires a dedicated spot in the home or office. This is because they generally weigh in the 30 to 40 lb. range.

Features to evaluate when looking for a desktop CCTV are:

1. Type of Monitor.

   The original monitors were like the original PC computer, a CRT (cathode ray tube). These are the large, bulkier screens. CCTVs with a CRT monitor, if they can still be found, are cheaper. Most monitors are the LCD (liquid crystal display), and are called flat screens. Within the LCD category are upgrades such as LED (light emitting diode) and TFT (thin film transistor). A LED is how the LCD screen is lit, and refers to having better contrast. TFT refers to something called active matrix LCD (AMLCD), meaning it reacts quickly to image changes (less blurring with movement). There is a more in-depth discussion about screen types at the end of this section.

   The larger the screen, the greater the field of view and the greater the for practical magnification. A 22 inch monitor will give a greater field of view enabling you to see more words with higher magnification rating than a 14 inch monitor.

2. Features of the Monitor.

   - Contrast/Brightness. There should be an adjustment for contrast/brightness, this is standard, and important for those with low contrast sensitivity or those who have problems with glare.
   - Magnification. There should be adjustment for various levels of magnification. The adjustment can be continuous (zoom) or jump by number. The range is usually something like 2x to 50x. Again, magnification capability varies by screen size.

- Focus. Focus can be manual, autofocus, or both. Both means that there is a manual override of the autofocus. This is desirable when working with three dimensional objects such as working on hobbies or repairs on small objects.
- Reverse Mode (reverse polarization). A CCTV with this capability can reverse black print on a white background to white print on a black background, and is also standard. Those with glare sensitivity will find it easier to view white letters on a black background.
- Color Option(s). It is nice to have natural or true color. This is good for viewing photos or any work where color is important. Some have the option of artificial colors, like yellow and black or blue and yellow, and likewise have reverse mode. (e.g. yellow letters on black background, or black letters on yellow background).

3. Make sure there is enough distance between the monitor and the table to give you the ability to use it as a writing surface.

   Here are some bells and whistles to evaluate:

   1. Ability to Adjust Monitor Height and Tilt of the Monitor. Some monitors are fixed in position. If not adjustable, you will need to find the right desk height and chair height to get the screen in a comfortable position for long-term viewing.

2. Manual Focus, Autofocus, or Both. Manual focus ability is desirable for viewing three dimensional objects.

3. Lots of other Font Color Options. This comes down to personal preference, not so much as need.

4. Computer Compatibility. This is the ability to attach to a computer. The manufacturer will also offer a split screen capability with this option.

5. Line Markers and Window Masking. These are features used to help the reader follow lines of text. The line marker is a line on the monitor window, centered to help guide your movement of the XY table beneath. Window masking is the darkening of the reading area above and below the line of text so as to 'highlight' the line of text.

6. Ability to Collapse for Storage. Usually it is just the monitor that folds down to give it a lower profile.

7. Text-to-Speech Capability. This is the capability of the CCTV to translate the printed word on the screen to spoken text.

8. Touch Pad Control is an upgrade that dispenses with the mechanical XY table and the feature control knobs. The user controls the options and moves the viewing area with finger movements on a touch pad.

Photos:

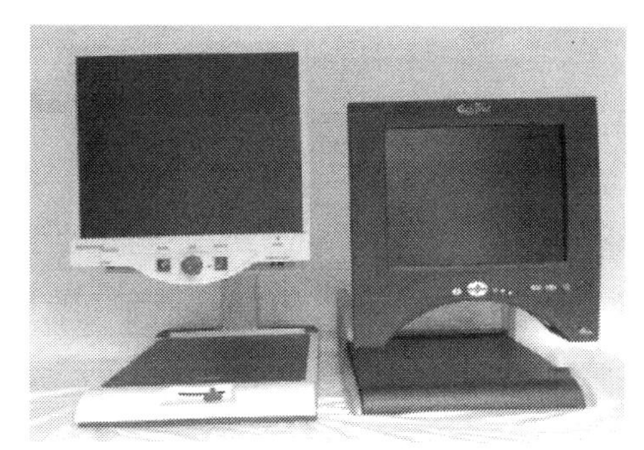

2 brands of Desktop CCTVs.

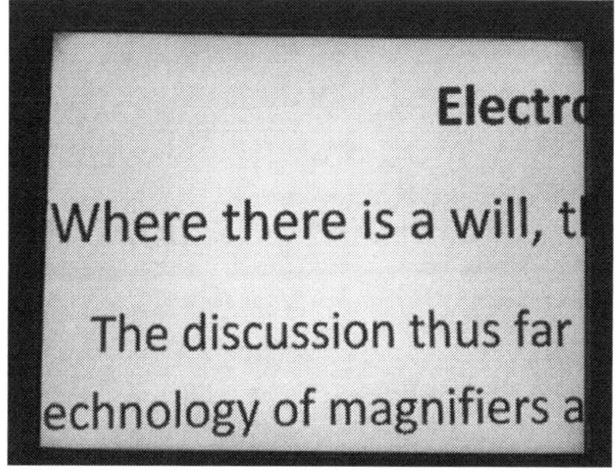

'Normal' black on white mode.

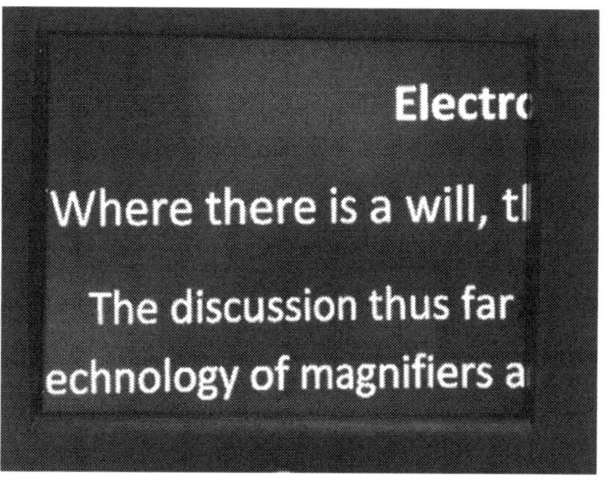

Inverse mode, white on black.

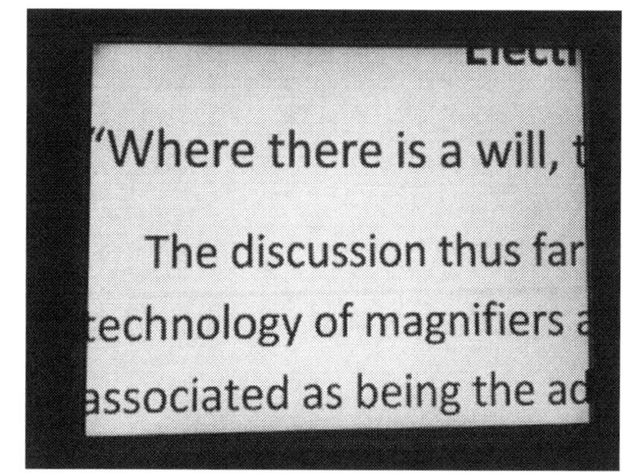

Line marking.

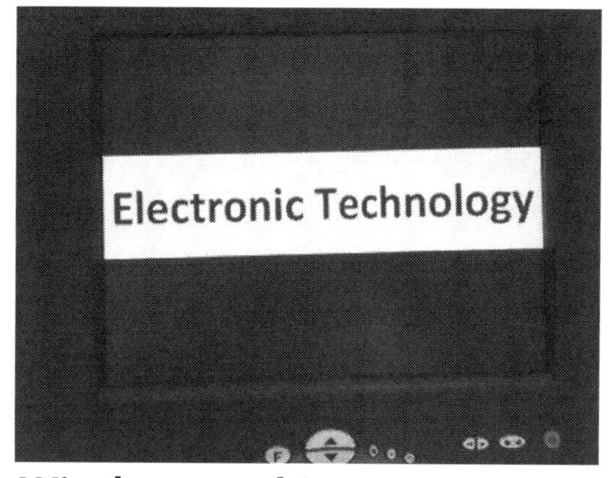

Window masking.

2. Portable Table Top CCTV.

This is the portable CCTV for school or work. There is no XY table, therefore it does not have the ease of reading that the desktop does. Portable CCTVs are a camera, either mounted to a monitor, or on a stand. The monitor is a flat screen LCD-type. There are 'portable CCTVs' that are sold as just the camera and control unit, which can then be attached to your own monitor or television.

Portables have the same standard features as the desktop: magnification adjustment, contrast/brightness control, reverse polarization, and additional screen color options.

What most (but not all) portable units offer, that the desktop CCTV does not, is a flexible camera mount. Because of this, the camera can be rotated to point at a distant object for viewing on the monitor. This is a great option for students in the classroom, or meeting attendees, to bring the distant presentation board closer and larger. Another use for the flexible camera is for self-viewing for grooming purposes. As much fun as it may be to try to get your foot on the XY table of your desktop CCTV to cut your toenails, it is not the easiest way.

Similar to the desktop CCTV, you should evaluate the magnification, color options, reverse modes, and contrast/brightness controls. Keep in mind, the larger the television or monitor, the greater larger the field of view for increased magnification capability.

A few other things to evaluate when looking at the portable CCTV are:

1. Monitors. These are included with most units, but not all. Evaluate the size of the monitor.

2. Weight. They generally weigh 9 lbs to 20 lbs (with the monitor). Units without a monitor will be about 1 to 3 lbs.

3. Manual focus, auto focus, or both.
4. Power Sources. Does it have the capability to run on rechargeable batteries, if no plug-in outlet is available? How long is the battery life?
5. Evaluate the Type of Camera Mount. Types are: suction mounts, camera attached to a flat panel base, and those mounted to a monitor. Check to see if the camera controls are on the camera mount or separate. Also, are the controls conveniently located and well demarcated by either color or tactile means?
6. Check the Flexibility of the Camera Mount for near, distance, and self-viewing. Not all portable units have the flexible camera feature. Those units that do not have a flexible head mount are only for reading.
7. Ease of setting up, storage, and portability.
8. Carrying case is included with some models, and for other models, it is an optional purchase.

Bells and whistles to look for are:

1. Computer Connectivity Compatibility. Capability to connect to a laptop computer, with additional hardware. This turns it into a laptop compatible video magnifier (covered in the next section);
2. iPAD or Android Tablet Connectivity. Tablet compatibility

makes it super portable by either a cable or wireless connection.

3. Capability for Optical Character Recognition (OCR) Scan and Text to speech (TTS). (these two features are explained in more detail later in this chapter);
4. Line Markers and Window Masking; and
5. A few models offer an XY table as an optional purchase.

3. Computer/Laptop Compatible Video Magnifier

When you purchase this technology, you are purchasing the camera, control unit, and the accompanying software to load on to your laptop computer. This unit will have contrast/ brightness control, the flexibility for near, distance, and self-viewing, and magnification adjustment (now called zoom). Keep in mind, the larger the laptop screen, the greater the field of view and capability for magnification.

Features to evaluate when buying a laptop compatible video magnifier are:

1. Manufacturers Specifications for Laptop Compatibility. Most all cameras require Windows XP or later or Mac OS X 10.8 or later. Check manufacturers specifications for type of processing unit and the amount of available memory (RAM) needed to run the camera and software. Also, there are some that require more than one USB port. Understand

that the better the laptop the better functioning the system will be.

2. Source of Power. The camera can run on either a plug-in wall adaptor, rechargeable battery, or off the power of your laptop. If it is battery, what is the battery life? Four hours seems average. Running on battery may get you through a few classes or lectures, but probably not through an entire day. Either an plug0in wall adaptor or spare batteries will keep the system running. If the camera runs off the laptop, it will run the charge on your computer at a faster rate.

3. Location of Controls. Evaluate where the controls for the system are located, and how much is controlled on the laptop keyboard.

4. Weight. The weight should be 5 lbs or less. Remember, you have to transport it along with your lap-top. A carrying case should be included. Once you get there, evaluate how easy will it be to set up.

5. Flexibility. Computer compatible camera units should have the flexibility for distance, near, and self-viewing. Check to see if the camera can be used on both sides of the computer. This maybe an important consideration for those who are left handed.

6. Near Viewing Lens. Look at where the lens for near viewing is located and how it is positioned when needed.

Some bells and whistles to look for include:

1. Screen Grabber Function. An image (say a slide presented on the board at a distance, or a page in a book), is 'freeze framed,' and then can be stored on the computer for future review.

2. Locator Finder Function. This feature can be used to zoom 'out', to locate that area of interest, and then zoom 'in' to magnify the details of that location. A large area is tedious to scan when looking for a particular part.

3. Split Screen Capability. This feature puts the material you are working with on your computer with the image viewed by the camera (distant or near). Keep in mind that your computer magnification software must be compatible with this feature.

4. Capability for Optical Character Recognition (OCR) Scan and Text to Speech (TTS). (These two features explained in more detail, later in this section.)

5. Line Markers and Window Masking. This feature help with following or isolating text to help with reading.

The combination of a top-of-the-line laptop computer, your magnifying software, and the portable camera system, turns out to be the most expensive of the video magnifier options. But it could be the most valuable system for students and the working visually impaired.

4. Hand-Held Video Magnifiers

Hand-held video magnifiers are the electronic equivalent of the hand-held and stand optical magnifiers. Likewise, these will be used for spotting and short term-use. The advantage of the electronic head-held magnifies over the hand-held optical magnifiers, is the larger field of view and variable magnification. Electronic magnifiers also have other useful features.

Similar to the larger CCTV, the hand-held video magnifier has a screen, camera, and a light source. Some of the features are the same. There is variable magnification, inverse mode, and full true color. The advantage is their portability and to be truly portable, it should come with a carrying case.

There are three general categories of hand-held video magnifiers:

1. Mini Hand-Held Video Magnifier is designed for pocket portability. They can be the size of a credit card or cell phone, and weigh about 4 oz. This video magnifier will be used for reading menus, checking price tags, and reading labels.

Some features to evaluate are:

1. Screen Size. The screens are small, in the 1.8 inch to 3.5 inch range. Check the quality of the screen. The display images should not have motion blur, as the magnifier is moved across the page. (also referred to as 'ghosting 'shadow-blur', shadow-trail.)

2. Magnification. There are usually about 3 or 4 choices for magnification ranging anywhere from 1.8X to about 18X. Remember, the small screen limits the field of view, and therefore the practical level of magnification. Reading two letters at a time at 18X mag is not practical.

3. Controls. Evaluate where the controls are for both visibility and ease of use. The controls are simple on/off, magnification, and freeze frame. The buttons should be visible by size, color, and/or tactile cues.

4. Viewing Options. Most have true color, black and white with grayscale options. Those that offer five or more mode options are offering other color choices with inverse modes. The most common color options are yellow and black, and yellow and blue.

5. Type of Battery, and Battery Life with Continuous Use.. Magnifiers should be good for two to three hours on a fully-charged battery. Replacing regular batteries will be an ongoing expense. Most use rechargeable batteries and should have an plug-in wall adaptor cord included to recharge the batteries by directly attaching to the magnifier, as opposed to pulling the batteries out to recharge.

6. Stand to Mount Magnifier for Extended Use. The advantage of the mini models is their small portable size, and not so much for long-term use. But a stand is a nice option.

Bells and whistles to consider are:

1. Auto shut off. This is a good battery-saving feature. It is set to turn off, on its own, if not moved for a period of time, say five minutes.

2. Adjustable Brightness Control. This feature is not absolutely necessary, but it is nice to be able to adjust screen brightness, especially in a dim restaurant so the magnifier doesn't turn into a beacon light in the room.

3. Ability to Turn Off the Magnifiers LED Light. This is helpful when viewing another screen, like a cell phone that has its own source of illumination.

4. Video Output. This will allow the mini to be attached to a TV monitor to amplify the magnification.

2. Standard Hand-Held Video Magnifier. These mid-sized video magnifier is still portable, but will fit better in a handbag or brief case. This type is a little bulkier because it will have a retractable handle by which it is used like a hand-held optical magnifier, or 'legs' that it stands on, like an optical stand magnifier, as it is glided across the page. This is a better option for the unsteady hand. This is by far the largest category of hand-held video magnifiers.

Some features to evaluate are:

1. Screen size. The screen size is slightly larger, at around 4

to 5 inches. Review the quality of the screen, looking for motion blur as it is moved across the page. see the section on premium screen features following this section.

2. Magnification. Magnification rating is a wide range from 1X to 22X. The magnification will be offered in a series of steps, say 3X - 5X - 7X - 10X, that would be four steps. Some will offer the magnification as continuous zoom, which means there is an option for all magnification levels in between.

3. Weight. These are less than one pound. A lightweight model is about 7oz.

4. Controls. Evaluate where the controls are located.. Controls vary from large well marked buttons on the top, or are controlled on the sides, and may have an on screen menu.

5. Viewing Options. True color, black and white high contrast with inverse mode, and artificial colors with inverse modes are typically featured. Most have five or more viewing modes.

6. Battery Type and Battery Life. Usually 2-3 hours of battery life when fully charged. Again, these should have rechargeable batteries, with a plug-in wall adapter cord.

7. Low Battery Indicator. This may be in the form of an audio signal, led lights, or an on-screen indicator.

8. Capability to Write Under the Magnifier. Check the distance beneath the magnifier to see if it can be used for check writing or other short-term writing tasks.

Bells and whistles to consider are:

1. Auto Shut Off to Save Battery Power. If it is not moved for a period of time, say 5 minutes, it will shut off on its own.
2. External Video Input. This option allows hook-up to a camera.
3. External Video Output. This option allows hook-up to a television or monitor for increased magnification.
4. Memory Card. This option is to save images freeze framed on the magnifier.
5. Adjustable Contrast and Brightness. This is a feature not likely to be found in the mini-type.
6. Distance Viewing. The magnifier can be held up, to magnify and bring closer, objects from across the room. There are those brands that can view even further away. This is a good option to use on the street for reading street signs in an area that are not familiar to you.
7. Reading Lines and Masking. A few models have reading lines and masking to aid in following text.

3. Large Hand-Held Video Magnifier. Although still portable, these larger units are bulkier, and are best for what I describe as a kitchen table magnifier. They are handy for reading the mail, reading recipes, and skimming the newspaper. These are also useful for short-term reading and writing tasks, where a portable CCTV would be nice, but not practical, such as filling out forms in an office, or a trip to the library. They offer some additional features the smaller hand-held video magnifiers do not have. The larger screen gives a larger field of view and greater capability for practical magnification, but is awkward to hold. These models will come with a stand, or some type of support system, designed to tilt and will have space beneath for writing.

Features to evaluate are:

1. Larger Screen. Screen size will be about 6 to 7 inches. Evaluate the quality of the screen as the magnifier moves across the page, looking for motion blur and look at the quality of the image using different types of reading material. Look for upgrade in screen quality. Some have evolved with HD (high definition = higher resolution) screens and blur-free technology (TFT).

2. Magnification. Magnification ranges from 3X to 26X (larger screen = greater practical magnification capability.) The magnification will be in steps or as continuous magnification referred to as zoom. The Zoom feature allows for magnification level control.

3. Weight. Generally they weigh over a 1 pound, and some are in the 2.5 lb range.

4. Controls. Similar to the other types of video magnifiers, evaluate location and ease of use. They should be easily

seen as large and/or colored, with tactile cues.

5. Viewing Options. Commonly, five or more mode options are offered, usually true color, black and white, high contrast black and white, blue and yellow, with inverse modes. Some offer more color options.

6. Type of Battery and Battery Life. When fully charged, the expected running time is about 4 - 5 hours. A plug0in wall adaptor and cord should be included for internal recharging.

7. Low Battery Indicator. This may be in the form of an audio signal, led lights, or an on-screen indicator.

8. Stand or Support System. Evaluate the flexibility of the screen tilt and the space available for writing beneath the magnifier.

Bells and whistles to consider are:

1. Auto shut off to save battery power. If it is not moved for five minutes, it will shut off on its own.

2. External Video Output. Some have the ability to attach to an external source. Attaching the magnifier output to a television or monitor can increase the field of view for magnifying.

3. Memory Card. This option is to save images freeze framed on the magnifier.

4. Brightness and Contrast Controls.

5. Distance Viewing. Capability to view not only near but distance targets. If it is held up, a clock across the room can be magnified and brought closer.
6. Reading lines and text masking. This is to help the user with page orientation and to follow lines of text when reading.

Photos:

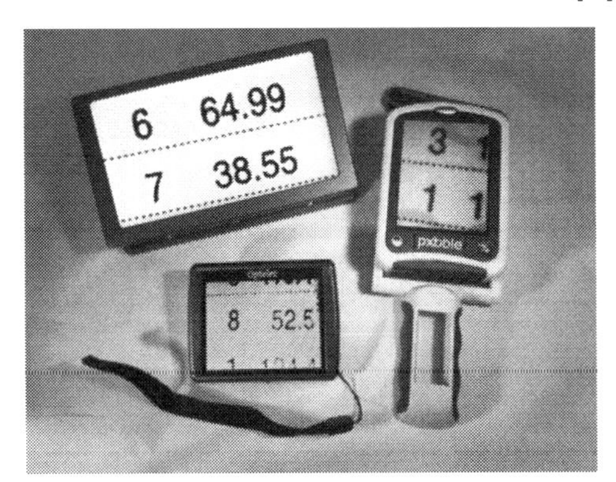

Large, standard and mini video magnifiers

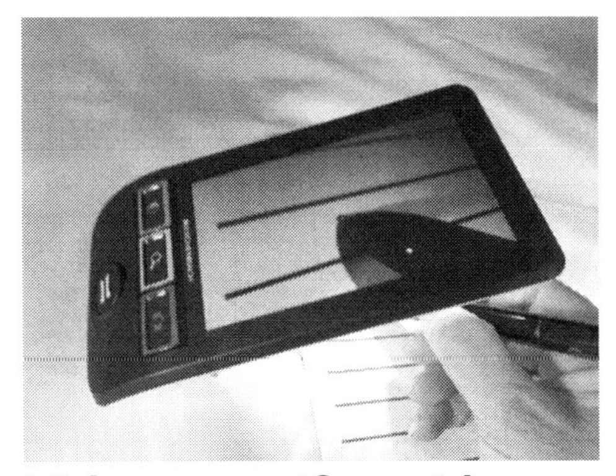

Video magnifier with stand allows for writing beneath

Hand-Held 'Mouse-Camera' Type Video Magnifier

This is generally not a portable type hand-held magnifier. It does look like a large computer-type mouse. The unit has a camera and a light source, and is attached to a monitor or television. So like the desktop CCTV, it will need a dedicated spot in the home or office. (There is always an exception. I did find a portable mouse-camera and monitor system). Considering the price of other video magnification systems, the combination of this unit with a monitor makes for a less expensive CCTV unit for reading, however lacking in options and flexibility.

Some of the features to look for are:

1. Magnification. The capability for magnification is dependent on the size of the monitor screen. Some of these units are fixed focus, meaning it has a set magnification size, and can be adjusted only by changing the size of the monitor screen.

2. Flexible Use. Evaluate if the unit can only be used on a flat surface, or if it can also be used on a curved surface (e.g. medication bottles, jars, cans).

3. Battery Type. Most have a rechargeable battery pack.

4. Color Options. Some models are only grayscale. Grayscale is the familiar old black and white televisions, where colors appear as shades of grey. Others offer true color

Some bells and whistles to consider are:

1. Magnification flexibility. A zoom feature will give a greater capability to increase or decrease magnification as needed.

2. Computer PC or Lap-top Compatibility. This is desirable if there is already a computer monitor available for use.

3. Wireless. Most are attached by a cable, but a wireless mouse magnifier can be found. This wireless type will have a plug-in wall adapter for recharging.

Monitors of CCTV and Video Magnifier:

Premium Features and Innovations

Monitor Types: CRT, LCD, and OLED

There are two commonly used types of monitors that desktop CCTVs utilize: the bulkier, older style cathode ray tube (CRT) and the flat screen liquid crystal display (LCD). The CRT monitor, like the CRT television, has fallen out of favor. As previously mentioned, desktop CCTVs with CRT screens are less expensive. These can be preferable over LCD monitors, because of better, truer color, and lack of motion blur.(1) An artist or graphic designer may find the CRT more desirable, where color is important.

The LCD monitor is thinner and lighter, takes up less desk space, and lends itself to the portable type of video magnifiers.

Another type of screen, often used with cell phones and smaller hand-held magnifiers, is the organic light emitting diode (OLED). OLED screens are more expensive.

Within the category of LCD and OLED screens there are premium features offered by manufacturers:

Premium Features of LCD and OLED Screens

Backlighting

There are two types of backlighting for LCD screens: cold cathode fluorescent tubes (CCFT) and light emitting diodes (LED). LCD screens that have LED lighting are desirable for better color and contrast, thinner LCD screens, lower power consumption (consider the size of the monitor), and no mercury, which means it is environmentally friendly and can be recycled.(2)

OLED screens do not have backlighting, and because of this it can have higher contrast and can be even thinner than LCDs. Currently OLED lit screens can be found in the more expensive mobile technology, particularly smartphones.

TFT

Thin film transistor (TFT) is a type of LCD screen called active matrix LCD (AMLCD) or a type of OLED called active matrix organic light emitting diode (AMOLED). Therefore, if 'AM' or TFT is not indicated that means that it is passive matrix LCD or OLED. The TFT is an additional layer to the LCD or OLED, to increase the speed, with greater image quality and contrast. It does this by determining how the pixels interact. Motion blur ('Ghosting 'shadow-blur', or shadow-trail) is slow pixel response.(1) The TFT option should help reduce the motion blur. (3)

High Definition

High definition is now appearing in manufacturers' product descriptions. LCD and OLED screens are a mass of 'pixels,' that is; 'picture elements,' of liquid crystals (neither liquid nor solid) or organic semiconductors (OLED).(3) High definition means they have crammed more pixels onto the screen, therefore giving the viewed image a higher resolution. Higher resolution allows more clarity of detail

The above-mentioned features, LED backlighting, OLED (organic semiconductors), TFT, and high definition, are implemented to solve the problems of contrast, motion blur, and resolution. Consider the quality of the screen and look for these features when selecting a CCTV/video magnifier. Consequently, as you can surmise, these premium features come at a higher price.

Optical Character Recognition (OCR) and Text to Speech (TTS)

These are not new technologies, but have an important application for the blind and visually impaired, especially students and those in the work force.

Optical Character Recognition (OCR)

Optical Character Recognition is a software program that 'translates' an image of text into computer electronic language. The camera or scanner attached to your computer is not 'reading' the text, but merely taking a 'picture'(camera) or 'capturing' (scanner) the image of the text. The OCR software processes the image by scanning the text presented to it, recognizing the characters (letters, numbers, and symbols) and organizing the electronic language so it can be manipulated by the user. The text can be saved, exported, e-mailed, edited, and/or highlighted. It can also be formatted into a MS Word, PDF, and html file. Font size, style, and color contrast modes can be selected. Reorganizing into readable text now makes it searchable.(4) The OCR may also be used with additional software for Braille output, magnification, MP3 formatting, or speech synthesization. These capabilities are dependent on which manufacturer's system you select.

Text-to-Speech (TTS)

The text to speech (speech synthesizer) software is one of the programs that can be combined with OCR to present text to the blind and visually impaired in audio format. There are two different OCR and TTS systems:

1. Hardware, also known as a stand-alone system; or
2. Software, which is loaded on to a compatible computer system.

Stand-Alone System (Hardware)

The self-contained hardware systems are commonly referred to as 'reading machines.' These tend to be the easiest systems for beginners, because of their right-out-of-the-box set-up. No computer experience is required. The simplest will read aloud books and documents. Others will have additional input and output capabilities. There should be a large button control panel, that controls voice, speed, and volume.

The text to be read is input into the system by way of a scanner. There are two types of scanners;

1. Flatbed or sheet fed scanner; and
2. Mounted camera.

Features to evaluate when selecting an OCR/TTS system are:

1. Speed. Speed with which the document is read. The simplest will do one page at a time; others can scan multiple pages while the user begins listening.

2. Voice Options. Some have better quality and natural sounding voices with two or more voice selections (male or female). The speed of reading may also be adjusted.

3. Weight. A complete system, which does not have a monitor, will weigh from 6 to 18 lbs.

4. Navigation. Navigation options allow the user to pause, rewind, or advance. Most have audio prompts for navigation cues.

5. Flexibility in the Types of Documents it can Read. Some will have difficulty with thick books, 3-dimensional items (cans, medicine bottles) or text written in columns. Only a few can read PDF files.

6. Language Options.

7. Storage Capacity. Simpler models will have maybe a 20-page memory, others have large storage capacity. One model, that has a large memory, also comes preloaded with books.

Bells and whistles to consider are:

1. Output. There are those that can be attached to a monitor or television. If attached to a monitor, the screen will display the text and highlight what is being read so the listener can follow along. Magnification and color modes, with an on-screen menus, can be modified. An outlet for headphones helps with privacy and doesn't disturb the library crowd. A

few models will attach to a Braille display for the blind.

2. Input Options. Those with a CD player can read audio formatted DASIY (digital accessible information systems) or the user can listen to music. A USB (input and output) port will enable flash drives for text and MP3 formats. Microphones can be used to input notes or markers by the user.

3. Additional Power Source. Stand-alone reading units are ac current powered. Those that can also run on battery power can be more portable.

4. Capability to Read Currency.

Computer OCR and TTS (software)

The software OCR and TTS in combination needs to be loaded onto a compatible personal/laptop computer. Like the computer compatible CCTV, there must be a compatible operating system, processor, RAM, and hard drive space. Most require a Windows OS. Macintosh OS compatible systems can be found. The OCR/TTS software requires a sound card, CD-Rom drive, keyboard, and compatible scanner. Make sure your computer system can support this software. This technology can put a powerful demand on the computer. Review the manufacturer's requirements before purchasing both software and scanner.(5)

Features to look for are similar to the stand-alone units. Consider voice sounds and available language options. This technology can be used for downloading books, magazines, and work-related material and for accessing electronic text formats available via the computer. The more sophisticated programs can also read PDF, HTML, MP3, DAISY, and scan the internet for e-books. Uploaded reading material can now be listened to, highlighted, edited, saved, and exported.

There are software screen reading programs, and there are magnifying programs, and then there are those that combine screen reading with screen magnification. Sellers will either sell a software compatible camera or scanner as a package, or offer one as an additional purchase.

Hand-Held Portable OCR/TTS Accessible Technology

These are the stand-alone smaller versions of the desktop 'reading machines.' The Aquos® is a hand-held magnifier that has OCR/TTS capability. The KReader Mobile® is the portable OCR/TTS best know, as a workhorse portable unit. It utilizes a digital camera as the scanner. Similar to the desktops, portable models have tactile control buttons with voice instructions and, additionally, have a screen for navigating and image placement (for capturing).

Images of the text to be read are taken by hovering the camera over the reading material. The on-board voice guides your placement of the camera. This small reader can capture a text image, save the image for later reference, and the saved information can be transferred to a personal computer. Portability makes it convenient for reading currency. The KReader also reads in multiple language, and even translates between languages. Headphones give privacy to what you are reading. These units run on rechargeable batteries.

There are Text-to-Speech apps for the cell phone that turns your device into a scanner/reader for greater portability and convenience. KNFB Reading Technologies has a Mobile Reader application for cell phones, which includes the Nokia phone with the Symbian S60 operating system and for the Apple iOS. It has many of the same capabilities as the KReader Mobile. It guides the user through the document scanning with voice and vibration. There is voice and on-screen navigation for document reading. Documents can be imported and exported. These apps read many document types and the apps can also store them. There are even more languages than the KReader Mobile, and can translate between them.

Personal Computer Accessibility (Desktop and Laptop)

The operating systems of desktop and laptop computers have included in their software applications, programs for accessibility. Accessibility features include customization options, not only for the visually impaired, but also for those with hearing, movement, and cognitive disabilities. This is good to know for those with multiple disabilities.

There are three aspects to making your computer more accessible:

1. Monitor. The first step for the print disabled is to get a larger monitor. Remember, as you magnify text, the field of view becomes smaller. The larger the monitor, the greater the potential for practical magnification because of the larger field of view.

You can customize your computer monitors by adjusting for brightness, contrast, and color temperature. Some flat screen televisions have the capability to be attached to computers. Keep in mind, however, a regular television on a desktop may lack the flexibility for you to change viewing angles.

2. Customize Settings. The second step is to customize operating system (OS) settings to optimize screen viewing for your vision.

   Personalization, or the ability to customize, allows you to change contrast, invert mode, grayscale, font, display settings, and other utility options. The cursor can be made bolder and the blinking rate changed. The mouse pointer shape and color can also be changed. These adjustments will make locating your position on a busy screen easier. It should be noted that not all operating systems offer these last mentioned pointer options.

   - Windows OS: The Control Panel opens up the Ease of Access Center (or Accessibility) and Personalization.
   - Mac OS X: Customization is done through the System Preferences and selecting Accessibility or Universal Access. Options can also be opened and controlled on the keyboard: Command + Options + F5.

3. Accessibility features. Next, familiarize yourself with the accessibility features of magnification, screen reading, and speech recognition applications, which are a part of the accessibility package included with your computer's operating system.

Operating System Screen Magnifiers and Screen Readers

The accessibility features included with computer operating systems provide for basic magnification and text-to-speech usage. The screen magnification and screen reader programs can be launched to enhance the viewing and navigation of other computer applications like web browsing, document reading, e-mail, and word processing. Look for these accessibility options under titles that include Accessibility, Ease of Access, Accessories, or System Preferences.

Each of these two applications allows for customization by the user. In the magnification utility, the user can adjust the amount of magnification and size of the magnified area. Different levels of magnification can be set for different software applications (e.g. email magnification vs. web browsing magnification size). Magnification mode choices include: the full screen, a lens (a magnified window that follows where the pointer goes), or docketed magnification (just a section of the screen is magnified, often found at the top of the screen), and/or split screen. Split screen mode magnifies half the screen, where the other half of the area is unmagnified. This helps with navigation, and is not available for all systems. Adjustments can also be made for brightness, contrast, and color reversal mode. Instead of black print on white background, invert to white letters on black background. I recommend this for anyone working on the computer in a dimly lit room.

Tip: Those that have a mild print disability can purchase a mouse with a 5X magnifier option. (Microsoft Optical Mouse) This mouse has a little thumb controlled button on the side, that when pressed, a magnifying 'lens' pops up on the screen. The pointer is the center of the 'lens,' and the lens follows where the pointer goes as you move it around the screen with your mouse. The size of the magnified area can be manipulated, the amount of magnification can be adjusted, and the colors can be inverted.

Screen readers are included as an accessibility feature. Essentially, the program reads aloud what is on the screen. Keep in mind that your system must have a sound card and speakers. The screen reader can be adjusted for speed, volume, and pitch. Some accessibility applications will have more than one choice of 'voices.' It takes some practice to learn to navigate with the screen reader. Warning: the magnifier and screen reader programs may not work simultaneously.

- Windows OS : Ease of access is where you can open up Narrator (screen reader) and Magnifier, or from the Start Menu type in Narrator. Magnifier can open up by pressing the Windows key and the + sign.
- Mac OS X: VoiceOver is launched through System Preferences >> Universal Access (or Accessibility) or from the keyboard: pressing Option + Command + F5 and the Zoom either from Universal Access or the keyboard, Option + Command + 8.

Operating System Speech Recognition Application

Speech recognition (also known as STT, speech-to-text) application has two functions: (1). Control of the computer activity by verbal commands, and (2). Dictation of text.

The commands to control computer activity are simple, but need to be learned. Things like open, page up, close, click, double click, reflect keyboard commands. Both Microsoft and Apple have tutorials to help you learn how to interact with your computer by a voice commands.

Voice recognition can also substitute for typing, such as word processing, email, and filling in the blanks in online forms. This is commonly called dictating. Accuracy is pretty good, but a review is a good idea to avoid silly looking mistakes. It helps to have a good quality microphone and good pronunciation.

- Windows OS: Speech Recognition is accessed through Control Panel>> Ease of Access>>Speech Recognition.
- Mac OS X: Dictation is accessed by way of System Preferences >> Dictation and Speech.

For all the above-mentioned accessibility features, there is usually more than one way to access them. Look for keyboard shortcuts to make accessibility features more accessible .

A shortcut to enlarge type when web browsing is to hold down the Ctrl button on your keyboard, and roll the scroll wheel on your mouse. You will see the entire screen enlarge. It will become larger as you scroll in one direction, and grow smaller in the other direction. (Windows)/ Mac OS X has a similar shortcut using the mouse or track pad. There are also keyboard shortcuts, for example: Ctrl + Plus sign (+) to zoom in, or Ctrl + Minus sign (-) to zoom out (Windows). Mac OS X systems have very similar function using the Option-Command keys and the + or - keys.

Third-Party Screen Magnification and Screen Reader Software

While the screen magnification and reader software included with your computer's operating system is fine for basic computer usage, those that need accessibility for work and education need a workhorse magnifying and screen reading solution. There are several options for the hard-core computer users. Those software packages can be purchased as either a stand-alone screen magnifier software or screen reader software, or purchased as a bundle. These software applications offer more flexibility in options, are more refined in personal customization, and offer high-quality performance versus the magnification and screen reading software included with your computers operating system. The magnified text will appear clearer, less pixilated with higher magnification, and therefore will be easier to read. The screen reader software will also have more voice choices that may be more natural sounding.

Third-party screen magnification and screen reading programs can be purchased as a CD format from a dealer or, in some cases, directly from the manufacturer. Programs can also be purchased as a download from the seller's website. Some manufacturers will offer a free trial from their website. Remember to check the software requirements for compatible operating system, processor, RAM, and hard drive space.

If portability is important, look for the capability to take the screen magnifying and reading program along with your customized settings in the form of a flash drive which can be loaded onto whatever computer you are using,, and then unloaded when you leave.

Speech Recognition Software (Speech-to-Text, STT)

There are also third-party software speech recognition programs. Speech recognition programs allow the user to give vocal commands and the ability to dictate text to the computer. The user may notice that the third-party software is more accurate.

The voice commands can be used to open other software applications. These commands are specific for the system, but are simple and somewhat intuitive. For example: Say the name of the key: "File," "Start," "Scroll." Commands can be in the form of an activity, for example: "Open" or "Switch to...," "Page up." There is a defined nomenclature to which the program responds.

Speech recognition software can also respond to the dictation of text into word processing, e-mail, and online forms. Although fairly accurate, you should always proofread the dictation.

In addition to the software, your computer will need to have a soundcard and microphone.

Feeling Computer Illiterate?

You are not alone! Questions may arise like: "This is all very nice, but how do I access these features, if this thing does not come with a manual?"(Manuals are so old school!) Most of the time, friends and family who use computers are not familiar with accessibility features, because they do not need to use them. Those of us, who have to figure this out for ourselves, need to know this: there is help out there, in the form of the internet. Manufactures of these operating systems have put their 'manuals' online. You can narrow your search by typing into the search engine (Google, Bing, Yahoo) bar what you are looking to do. For example:

'Access Mac OS Magnifier'

The search results that appear are choices for accessing that information, not only from Apple Accessibility websites, but forums and blogs of self-professed experts, and YouTube videos. Try asking a question:

'Why is the magnifier stuck at the top of the screen in Windows 7?'

Tech support web pages come up from Microsoft, along with web forum discussions and blogs. Note that it is important to indicate which operating system you are using (e.g. Windows Vista, XP, 7, 8,). There can be differences in options, features, and defaults between operating system versions.

Use tutorials where you can get them.

Type in to the search bar:

'Windows OS Accessibility tutorial.' What should come up:

Microsoft Accessibility: Technology for Everyone, Home

www.microsoft.com › enable

or to be more specific type in ' Windows 8 accessibility':

Windows 8 Accessibility Tutorials - Microsoft

www.microsoft.com › enable › training

Type in 'Mac OS Accessibility tutorial.' What should come up:
OS X Accessibility 101 - Tuts+ Computer Skills Tutorial
computers.tutsplus.com › tutorials

Head Mounted Electronic Low Vision Aids

The promise of portable head-mounted , hands free, low vision aids have been on the drawing board and as prototypes since the 1990s. There were a few that were made available for purchase, but, were met with limited success. This technology is now emerging as a viable innovation that is commercially available. Head mounted electronic low vision aids are more flexible and practical than earlier models.

Older technology, like the optical telescopes described in an earlier chapter, were designed primarily for spotting or reading, in a stationary position. Previous electronic technologies were rather large and weighty.

Basically, an electronic magnifying head borne low vision device is a CCTV on your head. There is a camera, a processing unit (probably on your waistband or in your pocket), and a screen. This technology has evolved over the past decade resulting in thinner lighted screens, and even smaller cameras with better resolution and focusing capabilities. Computer technology aids with object recognition and spatial orientation.

The advantages of a head mounted system are binocular viewing and hands free flexibility for activities of daily living. Factors to consider when reviewing head mounted low vision aids are:

1. Flexibility for Use of the System. Is the system designed for a particular activity, or will it allow for movement? Do you need to sit down to use it, or is it possible to walk around with it on? Consider your needs for the system. This includes not only reading, but also watching television, computer work, sporting events, and theater.

2. Flexibility of Functions. Evaluate the capability to customize features, such as magnification, brightness, and contrast control. Consider also the field of view.

3. Weight and Appearance. This may not seem important when talking about better vision. The reality is that it needs to be comfortable and feel natural for long-term use. My prediction is that whoever makes the most comfortable, normal looking head mounted aid will be the most successful.

4. Ease of Operation. A system that performs right out of the box (with maybe some instruction and practice) is preferable over a system that requires a weekend sabbatical to learn to operate it.

5. Cost. Currently, there are no inexpensive options. The range is about $3,500 (price of a desktop CCTV) to $15,000 (price of a late model used car).

Since there are only a few available in the market at this time, I will mention two by name.

eSight

These electronic glasses were developed by an electrical engineer, Conrad Lewis, to help his two sisters who have Stargardt's Disease. The electronic system magnifies and enhances vision.

eSight glasses are customized for the individual using prescription eyewear, in a carrier frame, over which the headset is mounted. The headset is comprised of a camera and an OLED screen (same thin and light, high resolution screen used by smartphones). This head mounted unit is attached to a compact computer processing unit by a cable. The processing unit and power unit are housed together. On the processing unit, the wearer can control the zoom magnification, brightness, contrast, color mode, and focus. eSight glasses can be used for distance viewing and focused up close for near. The headset allows the user to view a full screen magnification, or by tilting the headset up, the upper field can still be magnified, and the users unaided lower peripheral visual field can be used for walking around.

This is best suited for those with maculopathy and who still have residual vision. Although it can be beneficial for anyone who needs magnification, such as people with diabetic retinopathy, albinism, cone-rod dystrophies, LHON, and some forms of glaucoma and retinitis pigmentosa.(8)

There is a You Tube video titled ' How eSight Works.'

OrCam

Cam is for camera and Or means light in Hebrew. OrCam is an Israeli based company that has developed a wearable camera that attaches to the user's regular eyeglasses. It does not magnify or enhance vision as it does not have a screen. However, the system serves as an interface between what the user selects as a point of interest and an audio feedback to the user. The system utilizes recognition and reading software.

The camera unit and speaker unit clips onto the temple piece of any eyeglass frame, and is connected to the processing unit by a cable. The camera figures out what the user is looking at by means of a hand gesture. In this way the computer, by way of the camera, figures out what the user is interested in knowing about the scene, matches it to what is in its database, and then provides that information instantaneously. It provides this information through a bone conduction earpiece mounted behind the ear. It is also teachable, meaning it can learn to identify new objects. OrCam can be used to read text, identify signal lights, and object recognition.(9,10).

There is a You Tube video titled 'OrCam - See for Yourself.' and a TED talk, NYC Oct. 2013, Amnon Shashua presenting OrCam.

There are other research projects ongoing which utilize the newest technology to aid the visually impaired and the blind.

OpenGlass is a project that utilizes GoogleGlass technology as a platform for assistive technology. It promises innovative technology for recognition and mobility, by using an internet connection. (11)

Helpful websites:

- AbleData: Assistive Technology
  abledata.com
- AccessworldAmerican Foundation for the Blind
  afb.org
- Apple - Accessibility - OS X
  apple.com › accessibility
- Microsoft Accessibility - Technology for everyone
  microsoft.com › enable
- Windows - Microsoft
  windows.microsoft.com
- CNET Consumer technology information
  cnet.com

Resources:

Information on Technology from Manufacturers and their products, used as a resource for this chapter:

CCTV

- Enhanced Vision**www.enhancedvision.com**
  - Merlin
- Eschenbach Optik **www.eschenbach.com**
  - MagniLink
  - Presto Life (Ash Technologies)

- Freedom Scientific **www.freedomscientific.com**
    - Topaz
- HIMS Inc. **www.hims-inc.com**
    - Lifestyle HD
- Humanware **www.humanware.com**
    - Prodigi and Prodigi Duo
- MagniSight **www.magnisight.com**
    - Explorer
- Optelec **us.optelec.com**
    - ClearView
- Telesensory **www.telesensory.com**
    - Aladdin
    - Sunshine Pro (CRT monitor)

Portable Desktop Magnifiers

- The Chicago Lighthouse **http://chicagolighthouse.org/**
    - DaVinci HD Talking CCTV
- Enhanced Vision **www.enhancedvision.com**
    - Acrobat
- Eschenbach Optik **www.eschenbach.com**
    - MagniLink
    - Eclipse Touch Scholar 2 (Ash Technologies)
    - Prisma
- Freedom Scientific **www.freedomscientific.com**
    - Topaz PHD

- Onyx

- HIMS **Inc.www.hims-inc.com**
  - E-bot
  - Sense View DUO
- Humanware **www.humanware.com**
  - Smartview 360
  - Prodigi Connect 12
- Optelec **us.optelec.com**
  - Optelec MultiView
- Telesensory **www.telesensory.com**
  - Vertex

Computer / Lap top Compatible Magnifiers (Hardware)

- The Chicago Lighthouse **http://chicagolighthouse.org/**
  - Flick
- Enhanced Vision **www.enhancedvision.com**
  - Transformer
- Eschenbach **Optikwww.eschenbach.com**
  - MagniLink S
  - Opti Verso 2 (Ash Technologies)
- Optelec **us.optelec.com**
  - ClearNote

Hand-Held Video Magnifiers

- Bierley Electronic Magnifiers **www.bierley.com/**
  - Explora

  - Explora-Plus
- Enhanced Vision **www.enhancedvision.com**
  - Amigo
  - Pebble and Pebble Mini
- Eschenbach Optik **www.eschenbach.com**
  - Mobilux Digital Touch HD
  - Smartlux
  - Crystal XL (Ash Technologies)
  - Quicklook (Ash Technologies)
- Freedom Scientific **www.freedomscientific.com**
  - Ruby
  - Sapphire
- HIMS Inc. **www.hims-inc.com**
  - Candy HD
- Humanware **www.humanware.com**
  - Prodigi Tablet
  - Smartview Versa
- MagniSight **www.magnisight.com**
  - Looky+
- Mattingly Low Vision **www.mattinglylowvision.com**/
  - Mattingly SMART
  - SNOW 4.3″ and 7″
  - Eye-C
  - Aukey Ultra
- Optelec **us.optelec.com**

    - Compact HD
    - Traveller HD

- Telesensory www.telesensory.com
    - Pico
    - Olympia

Mouse-TypeVvideo Magnifier

- Enhanced Vision www.enhancedvision.com
    - Max

- Mattingly Low Vision www.mattinglylowvision.com/
    - Mattingly Wired Mouse

- Bierley Electronic Magnifierswww.bierley.com/
    - Momomouse
    - Colormouse
    - MPD-12 (mouse and screen combo)

OCR and TTS Hardware

- Ai Squared www.aisquared.com
    - ZoomText ImageReader (software and camera)

- Enhanced Vision www.enhancedvision.com
    - Smart Reader (stand-alone unit)
    - DaVinci (CCTV magnifier with OCR and TTS)

- Freedom Scientific www.freedomscientific.com
    - OPENBOOK and Pearl (software and camera)
    - SARA (stand-alone unit)
    - Eye-Pal Vision (stand-alone unit)

- Issist **issist1.com**
  - ReadDesk (camera + Windows comp. software)
- Optelec **us.optelec.com**
  - Clear Reader + (stand-alone unit)
- Plustek **plustek.com**
  - Plustek Book Reader V100 (stand-alone unit)
- Telesensory **www.telesensory.com**
  - Ovation (stand-alone unit)

Windows OS and Mac OS both have on-board magnifying and screen reading accessibility software. The following software can be purchased for more accessibility options and flexibility:

Third-Party Magnifying Software with Screen Reader

- Ai Squared **www.aisquared.com**
  - Zoom Text Magnifier/Reader (Windows)
  - Zoom Text for Mac (Mac OS)
- Dolphin Computer Access Inc **www.yourdolphin.com**
  - Supernova (Windows)
- Issist **issist1.com**
  - iZoom (Windows)

Third-Party Screen Reading Software

- Claro Software Ltd **www.clarosoftware.com**
  - ClaroRead (Windows, Reader and Writing)
  - ClaroRead for Mac

- Dolphin Computer Access Inc. **www.yourdolphin.com**
  - Guide (Windows)
- Freedom Scientific **www.freedomscientific.com**
  - JAWS (Job Access with Speech), (Windows)
- Kurzweil Education **www.kurzweiledu.com**/
  - Kurzweil 1000 (software for Windows)
  - Kurzweil 3000 (software, Windows or Mac OS)

Third-Party Magnification software

- Ai Squared **www.aisquared.com**
  - Zoom Text Magnifier (Windows)
- Freedom Scientific **www.freedomscientific.com**
  - Magic (Windows)

Portable Hand-Held OCR/TTS

- KNFB Reader **www.knfbreader.com** › products-mobile
  - KReader Mobile
  - KNFB Mobile Reader for iOS & Symbian (software)

Portable Hand-Held Magnifier with OCR/TTS

- Issist **issist1.com**
  - Aquos (magnifier and reader)

Speech Recognition Software

- Nuance **www.nuance.com** › dragon
  - Dragon Dictate- Naturally speaking (Windows or Mac OS)

Head Mounted Technology

- eSight Corporation **www.esighteyewear.com**
    - eSight
- OrCam Technologies **www.orcam.com**
    - OrCam

References

1. Steer, William Andrew, Phd, LCD monitor Technology and Tests. 3 Dec. 2011, 222. Retrieved from **techmind.org/lcd**/.
2. Franklin, Eric, Monitor Buying Guide. 21, Nov. 2013, Retrieved from **reviews.cnet.com/monitorbuyingguide/** .
3. Learn about LCD TV and TFT LCD displays. Retrieved from **www.plasma.com/classroom/What_is_tft_lcd.htm** .
4. Wenberg, Koert, Kendrick, Deborah, Levanthal, Jay. Recognizing and Rewording. A review of OPRNBOOK and Kurzweil1000. *Accessworld,* Sept. 2004.
5. Hodges, Brad, More than One Way to Read: A Review of Kurzweil 1000 and Openbook. Accessworld, Ju ly 2006. Retrieved from **http://www.afb.org/afbpress/pub.asp?DocID=aw070405**
6. Rempel, John, The Bigger Picture: A Comparative Review of Magnifier for Windows 7 and Zoom for Mac OS. Accessworld, March 2012, Volume 1, Number 3.
7. Hodges, Brad and Huffman, Lee. Screen Reading Alternatives: A Review of Lower Cost Options. AFB Accessworld, March 2009, Vol. 10, Number 2.
8. ESight Corporation. Website, **www.esighteyewear.com** FAQs.
9. Shashua, Annon. TED @NYC Oct 2013. Annon Shashua presenting OrCam.

10. Rich Shea. The OrCam Device; Giving Back Functionality. Eye on the Cure, Foundation Fighting Blindness, July, 17, 2013.

11. Duffy Maureen. Google Glass Applications for Blind and Visually Impaired. VisionAware Blog, Aug. 21, 2013. Retrieved from **www.visionaware.org**>blog

CHAPTER 16

Mobile Accessibility

Mobile accessibility is a feature of hand-held devices, such as cell phones and tablets, which makes mainstream communication available to those with impairments. But for those with visual impairments it can be more than just a means of communication. These mobile devices can be used as a tool for interacting with your surroundings. Information, by way of accessibility software applications, can be used to enlarge and give audio feedback to make print accessible, to enhance mobility, and to identify places and things.

The beauty of mobile technology is that it is designed for use by the masses, and because of that their use is very straight forward. There is an initial set-up, then you learn how to access features by way of hand gestures, and how to use carefully selected, accessibility features.

Although there are some phones which are specifically designed for the visually impaired and blind, off-the-shelf mobile devices can be configured for use by the disabled. No special orders or special pricing required.

Cell Phone Accessibility

Cell phone technology and how we use mobile devices is changing by leaps and bounds. If you are just looking for a basic communication device, there are phones designed for people who need a keyboard and basic phone access, without all the bells and whistles. If you look around at the various cell phone carriers, there are three general types:

1. Basic, big button cell phone;
2. Feature cell phone; and
3. Smartphone.

<u>Accessibility of the Basic Big Button Cell Phone</u>

The most accessible of the basic phones are those with the big buttons. The keypad has tactile buttons with large, high contrast, sometimes colored, printed numbers. The screen of the basic models is usually small, about two inches; and should be a bright display with good contrast. The numbers on the screen can be set to a larger font.

A few other features of the basic big button phones are:

1. A programmable phone book for contacts;
2. Text messaging capability;
3. Enhanced speakers for the hearing impaired;
4. Battery life when in use of about 3 to 7 hours; and

5. Those marketed to seniors will have an emergency response system and/or preprogrammed emergency call buttons. One carrier has an operator service available for purchase monthly to assist with making calls.

Additional bells and whistles features are,

1. Audio cues, and keys that speak;
2. Voice dialing from the programmed list of contacts;
3. Camera is found on a few, video capability is rarer;
4. FM radio;
5. Flashlight; and
6. Bluetooth capability for connectivity to headsets or speakers.

Feature Cell Phones Designed for the Visually Impaired

Feature phones fall in between basic phone and smartphones. Within the feature phone category there are those which are more highly evolved low vision accessible devices, although many off-the-shelf feature phones have some accessibility features. Those designed for low vision have large tactile buttons with accessible features, including audible cues and speaking text. The screens, although still small (palm size), have large font displays.

Features of the phones designed for low vision accessibility include:

1. Speaks everything on the screen. It will read the screen menu and list of contacts;

2. Speaks the keys as they are pressed;
3. Speaks caller ID and customizable ringtones;
4. Voice activated dialing from your list of contacts;
5. Speaks time and date;
6. Customization features for the screen, such as changing font size, brightness, contrast, and inverse mode (white print on black background); and
7. Programmable emergency numbers and alerts.

Additional features to consider are:

1. Text to speech for reading text messages;
2. Voice recognition ability to dictate text messages;
3. Languages choices available;
4. Internet access and web browsing; and
5. Camera with photo storage.

The Smartphone

Smartphones are powerful computers that you can hold in your hand. Not only are they a telecommunications device, but they are also a web browser, camera, media player for music and videos, book reader, clock, and portable inbox. The possibilities are almost endless. This is a tool that can be purchased 'off-the-shelf,' and does not need to be purchased at special low vision center.

Designers of software applications have addressed some of these accessibility issues by developing screen readers and magnification software to work in conjunction with various operating systems. But understand, not all off-the-shelf smartphones are created equal in this respect. Some come pre-loaded with accessibility features, and some are better than others. The individual phone service carriers will decide which phones will have certain accessibility features.

Filling the void are third-party software developers, who create software applications (commonly known as 'apps') that users can download to their smartphone. The smartphone can be an awesome tool for the visually impaired with the accessibility features in place.

Here's the issue - it can be daunting to select the best system for you, setting your accessible format, and learning to use it effectively and efficiently. Those of us who are not 'techies' can find the lingo and abbreviations confusing. There is also a learning curve as to hand gestures, finger tapping, and finger swiping, which can take a little practice.

For those who have difficulty seeing the screen, there are smartphones specifically designed for the blind and visually impaired (eyes-free technology). Those smartphones will have a simpler interface for ease of access and very straight forward features combined with auditory cues. They are preloaded with additional accessibility applications, such as: object recognition, currency and color identification, GPS, and ebook reading. There are added features of easy access for remote assistance to connect with operator assistance or family and friends to aid in object identification, navigation, and phone locater.

The basic operating systems (OS) for smartphones are: Windows (Microsoft), Android (Google), iOS (Apple), Blackberry (Blackberry), and Symbian (Nokia). These are not the only ones, but are the most common. Accessibility features for the operating system, may vary by the version (indicated by numbers 1.0, 2.0, or letters ce, xe, or some clever name etc.). The OS is an important consideration when choosing a phone or tablet. Keep in mind, accessibility features vary by smartphone model, and available apps vary by operating system.

Accessibility Features

Font Settings

Most phones, whether it is a basic, feature, or smartphone, allow for adjustment in the size and color of the print. Where they differ is how large the print can be made and the screen size. Brightness of the screen is another variable to enhance the screen by increasing contrast.

Color Inversion

This setting allows you to change black-on-white print to white-on-black print. Good for reducing glare, and I find good for reading in lower light levels in the evening. The inversion will also change the colors of everything else, such as: orange will appear blue, red appears green.

Text-to-Speech (Screen Readers)

The simplest form of mobile text-to-speech (TTS) will sound out the key numbers or letters as you touch them. The screen reader vocalizes what is under the user's finger. The choice is made when the user taps the icon, letter, number, or menu selection. Others will read aloud the caller id, contacts phone list, and menu options, which is very helpful for navigating through the features. A step above that are those that read on-screen print from text message, e-mail, books, and web pages.

Screen Magnifiers

Full screen magnifiers have variable levels of magnification to enhance viewing of the screen (frequently called zoom). There are some applications, like web browsing, where the screen can be enlarged by hand gestures such as taping, or the pinch open and pinch close hand gesture. Keep in mind, the larger the magnification, the smaller the area of the image that can be viewed.

Many smartphones come with a pre-loaded screen reader and may be bundled with magnifying software. Examples include:

Screen reader (TTS)		Magnifying SoftWare
Talks	plus	Zooms (Nuance)
VoiceOver	plus	Zoom(iOS)
MobileSpeak	plus	MobileMagnifier (Windows)

A suite, or bundle, of accessibility applications may be included as a part of the phones standard set of software apps, or it can be downloaded as a suite of accessibility features. Besides a screen reader and magnifier, the suite may include voice recognition (speech to text applications) and intelligent software assistant (voice activated commands).

Voice Recognition (VR)

This software is the opposite of text-to-speech. It turns speech to text. This application has the ability to type out text messages, e-mails, and type search key words into a web browser simply by speaking into the phone when the application is activated. This makes the task of typing easier on small, difficult to see, touch screen keypads.

Intelligent Software Assistant

This is a form of voice recognition that performs requested tasks. An intelligent software assistant allows you to give commands to your phone, to call contacts, or open a software application. Most notably it is useful for web searches, to answer straightforward questions (a name, a place, a sports score, etc.), or display search engine results. It is also useful for opening apps, without searching for the icon.

Tablets

This is similar to a smartphone in a book size format. Meaning they have the same capabilities, and the same setting features of the mobile phone operating system, but are not a traditional telecommunication device. It can, however, be used with downloadable, less traditional video-chat applications.

Tablets have the advantage of the larger screen; therefore magnified text will have a larger field of view. Many of the software applications available for a mobile phone are also available for a tablet with the same operating system.

In the chapter on the internet and information systems, tablets are discussed as an important tool for accessing information.

Apps (Software Applications)

Apps are software programs that enhance the functioning of other software (e.g., screen magnifiers), or add a new function to your phone or tablet (e.g., social networking). Many of the apps run through an internet browser, accessing data and media in a smartphone or tablet-friendly format. Smartphones and tablets come pre-loaded with functional apps, such as clocks, calculators, note books, calendars, games, and of course, access to purchase more apps.

Each operating system has their own store(s) for purchase of third-party apps. There are thousands of apps that give access to almost anything you can think of; but not all are created equal. There are a lot that are free and you can try them out. You will notice that some of these free apps will run advertisements, so that you will purchase the better, more user-friendly premium version. The more advanced programs will cost you. That is how they make their money.

Here are a few key words when looking for apps: accessibility, low vision, visually impaired, and blind. The number of available apps can be overwhelming, especially if you are not sure how it can work for you.

There are a few things you can do:

1. Read the reviews listed on each app page from the store. This is moderately helpful. This is someone else's opinion, and may not necessarily be the same experience that you have.

2. Some app developers have an off-store webpage for their app. Scroll down to 'Developers website.' Occasionally this is helpful for outlining the features of the app, and any purchases that can be made within the app.

3. Take it to the web browser. Often the app store lists too many selections, some are seemingly unrelated. Type into the search engine bar the type of app you are looking for. Names of individual apps will appear, and frequently, 'Top Ten ' lists or blogger discussions about particular apps. If you type in the words 'for the visually impaired,' the results will be more specific. For example: if you type in 'navigation app,' many results appear. But if you type in 'navigation app for the visually impaired,' a very few specific app listings will be listed.

4. Finally, you can try downloading the free or sample version and give it a try. This way you can understand the limitations, discover any 'in app' purchases, and keep the heroes and delete the zeros.

App Products to look for:

Magnifiers	OCR	CCTV
GPS	Navigation	Mobility
Money reader	Games	Color identifier
Note taking	Organization	Word processing
Radio	Podcasts	Music
Books	Newspapers	Magazines and more!

Personal Digital Assistants (PDA)

Personal digital assistants were originally designed as palm-sized organizers for people on the go. The advent of the smartphone with its multiplicity of software applications has dwarfed the PDA market. There are PDAs designed specifically for the blind and visually impaired to serve in education and business.

The PDA is a portable personal computer with voice output. Key features include contact list, calendar for appointments, web browsing capability, e-mail, media player, note taking ability with word processing, all with voice output. PDAs can be synchronized with the personal computer (desk or laptop) to keep data organized and updated.

It differs from a smartphone in that those designed for the blind and visually impaired have a keyboard for note taking, utilizing the tactile keys. The user accesses data on the PDA through the voice output, standard printer, or Braille output. Other accessibility features include DAISY format reading ability and voice recognition for note taking (speech-to-text).

Resources

Phones Designed for the Visually Impaired

- Assistech **assistech.com**
    - Snapfon ezTWO (Basic, big button phone)
- GreatCell **www.greatcall.com**/ (carrier)
    - Jitterbug 5 (Basic big button phone)
    - Jitterbug Touch 3 (Smartphone)
- Independent Living Aids, LLC **www.independentliving.com**
    - Just5 (Basic big button phone)
- Odin Mobile **odinmobile.com**/
    - ODIN VI (Feature phone)
    - Emporia Essence (Basic/Feature phone)
    - Emporia CLICK (Basic big button)
- RAY Project (eyes-free technology) **www.project-ray.com/**
    - Ray N5 (Google Nexus 5, Android smartphone)
    - Ray G1 (Huawei 510 smartphone)

Information on Accessibility Apps

AppleVis	**www.applevis.com** (Apple)
LookTel	**www.looktel.com** (Apple)
Ray app	**www.project-ray.com** (Android)
Disability apps	**www.appcessibile.org** (Apple and Android)

Personal Digital Assistants

- Humanware **www.humanware.com**
  - VoiceMate Apex QT
- Freedom Scientific **www.freedomscientific.com**
  - PAC Mate Omni

Other Resources

Apple – Accessibility – iPhone – Vision. Retrieved from **www.apple.com/accessibility/ios/**

Burton, Darien, Huffman, Lee. Dialing Up the Magnification: A Review of mobile Magnifier. AFB Accessworld Magazine, November 2005 Issue, Volume 6 Number 6

Dolcourt, Jessica., Souped-up Huawei Vision gives insight to the blind. June 5, 2013 3. Retrieved from **www.cnet.com**

Personal Digital Assistance &Speech. American Federation for the Blind . **www.afb.org**/ Home> Product Search> Browse by Category

iPhone, iPad and Android Apps for the Blind and Visually Impaired. *Date Posted: April 16, 2014* Retrieved from **Appccessible.org**.

Smartphones for Blind / Cell Phones for Visually Impaired. Retrieved from **www.project-ray.com/**

Using Google products – Accessibility – Google, Retrieved from **www.google.com/accessibility/products/**

Van Gerven, Clara. Odin VI Mobile Phone. National Federation of the Blind. Blog post January 13, 2014. Retrieved from **nfb.org**

CHAPTER 17

The Information Highway: The Internet and Beyond

Thus far, I have discussed ways of making standard print material accessible. Those options include magnification by optical devices, electronic magnifiers, and computer software applications for magnification, optical character recognition (OCR) and text to speech (TTS). There are other options for reading books, newspapers, magazines, and documents formatted for the print disabled and the blind.(1)

Formats and Technologies

Large Print

The first option that comes to mind for those with print disabilities is large print. Even with all the other options available, large print is still alive in the general marketplace and in education. Large print books can be found in the large print book section of libraries. Booksellers, both stores and online, have a wide selection of large print books, including bestsellers. Magazines, such as Readers

Digest, Guidepost and other faith-based magazines, can be found in large print, but there are not many of them. The New York Times newspaper produces a large print weekly edition, which is available for home delivery.

The standards for large print publications have been established by organizations for the blind and visually impaired along with those in the publishing industry.(2, 3) The National Association of the Visually Handicapped and the American Printing House for the Blind have taken leadership roles in establishing standards for large print. Recommended standards include recommendations of font type (a straight up and down style), font size (18 point), adequate spacing between lines of text (crowded text is difficult to read), and adequate margins. There are also recommendations for paper color, book size, and thickness. Nothing says visually disabled like carrying around a bestselling book the size of the world atlas.

Large Print: e-Books and e-Readers

Electronic books (e-books) are the digital form of text and images accessed through electronic devices. Electronic readers (e-readers) are a mainstream technology that the print disabled can customize to make any available e-book into large print. More developers of e-readers have entered the marketplace and the prices have come down substantially from when the Kindle was first introduced in 2007.

E-Readers are used to download books, magazines, newspapers, and blogs by wireless networks. No computer required! The user is able to access the developers own bookstore (Amazon, Barnes and Noble, Sony, Apple, Kobo) right from the e-reader screen. A user can also access books from their public library by way of the device. (See the discussion in this chapter, The Local Library and Overdrive).

The great advantage is that any available book can be a large print book at the same price as what everyone else is paying for reading material. Not only that, but e-books can be less expensive than the regular bound paper type (save a tree!) Additionally, e-readers have become so thin and lightweight; they are easier to handle than paperbound books, making them very portable in handbags and pockets.

E-book readers can typically be loaded with hundreds or thousands, of books, magazines, and newspapers, ready at your fingertips to be read. Most support the ePUB format, which is the open standard for digital text. The exception is Amazon Kindle, which uses a proprietary format: Mobi. Other functions are available; making them useful in other ways. The built-in dictionary is a useful feature. This gives e-readers an advantage over paper bound books as readers have the ability to look up words in the middle of reading.

Features to consider when purchasing an e-reader are:

1. Screen Size. Typically they are in the 6 to 7 inch range. This is a measurement taken on the diagonal. Smaller may seem better for portability, but consider, the smaller the screen and the larger the print, the fewer words visible on the screen when

the print is enlarged. A tablet, which can also be used as an e-reader, is usually around 9 inches on the diagonal.

2. Screen Type. There are the familiar backlit LCD and AMOLED type screens of tablets and cell phones. Then there are the e-ink or e-paper screens. These screens simulate paper in what is called a grey scale.(4) LCD screens are the higher contrast black on white and generally have color capability. The great benefit of the simulated paper screen is the ability to read outdoors. Anyone who has ever tried to read an LCD cell phone screen outdoors knows how difficult it can be. Although good for reading outdoors, the 'paper' screen requires good lighting to view comfortably indoors. Evaluate the contrast or lack of contrast of this type of screen. A premium feature of e-ink 'paper' screens is the addition of a built-in light for evening reading. Whereas, the LCD screen has a bright background, is good for contrast, but is bad for creating glare. The choice of backlit LCD or a 'paper' screen is a matter of personal preference.

3. Font Enlargement and Font Style. An e-reader may have a few font size choices, or can have a wide variety of choices. The maximum size depends on the reader unit. The sizes will have numbers like 1,2,or names like large or extra large. Therefore you are not able to determine font size and really have no idea what size 'Extra Large' will be. The best option is to watch a demonstration of changing font size to determine if it is adequate for your needs.

E-readers will often offer several choices of font styles, some of which may be easier to read than others.

4. Ease of Navigation. Doing away with keyboards and using touch screen controls has made the devices lighter and more compact. Unfortunately, but not unusual, the size of the font on the menu screens and icons cannot be adjusted and can be very difficult to read.(5) Look for audio navigation. This can be very helpful for the small print on the menu and option screens where the font size cannot be customized.

5. Internet Connection. Most connect exclusively by WiFi for access to the bookstore and for downloading. Some have the ability to also connect by 3G or 4G, which is the same wireless signal used by cell phones. This is a great option if there is no WiFi available. Keep in mind, however, there may be data use charges for downloading with the 3G or 4G connections.

6. Battery Life. Incredible claims are made. Most claims are in the 14 to 60 day range (e-ink screens).(6) These are the e-ink and e-paper screens, because they use less energy than LCD and AMOLED. The caveat is that the battery life, before a recharge is needed, depends on how the reader is used. Browsing, downloading, and reading literature with pictures will drain the battery sooner.

Bells and Whistles to look for in an e-reader are:

1. Contrast and Brightness Control. Interestingly, this is a specialized

feature for e-readers. A few have the ability to control the brightness of the menu screen, but if the printing is small, it may not be a significant advantage,.

2. Ability to Bookmark, Highlight Text, and Add Notes. Most e-readers have these options. Notes can be made by a pop up keyboard or an electronic stylus.

3. Ads, also known as. Special Offers. Watch for this additional feature. Ads do not come up in the text of a book, but will appear when you turn on the unit or when browsing. This option may not be entirely objectionable, if you are looking for bargains. Some will offer the ability to opt out of 'special offers,' for a price.

4. Memory Card Slot. The ability to use an SD memory card will expand available storage space for downloading text.

5. Page Numbers. This option comes in handy, especially when you are enlarging print. Otherwise you have no idea what page you are actually on. It might become important for referencing passages for your own interest or when conversing with others if you are in a book club.

6. Speakers and Headphone Jack. These two options make it possible to download and listen to audio books.

7. Text-to-Speech. This option turns a downloaded book into an 'audio' book. The voice, however, will not be as pleasant to listen to as the professionals who read for the true audio books. There

is a premium price to be paid for those professionally produced audio books.

Other options for reading books electronically are:

PC and lap top computers, smartphones, and tablets can all have e-books downloaded. Booksellers have 'apps' that when downloaded to your device, become the gateway for downloading reading material. Within the app, there are options for customizing for your personal reading needs. Smartphones, because of their small screens, are obviously not a good choice for large font size.

The larger screen e-readers have more in common with tablets, like web browsing, e-mail, color LCD screens, and third-party applications like games.(7) These tablet e-readers are a little bulkier, heavier, and understandably more expensive.

Audio Players and Formats:

Compact Disc (CD) Players

The CD player is a familiar, yet older technology, that most people have in one form or another. They can be found as a portable unit or part of a computer system, a home stereo system, a radio unit, and commonly are found in cars. Portable units are relatively inexpensive. Those who demand good audio quality will find that CD players offer the best. Those are the advantages.

The disadvantage is that CD players can be more difficult to navigate through text. Like most mainstream technology, the option and control buttons and digital screen readout is most likely small font and can be difficult to read. The screens tend to be exceedingly small, with minimal information. Some players lose your place when you turn them off. So you need a good memory to find your place at the beginning of that chapter. Look for the auto-resume option to get around this problem. If the portable unit does not have anti-skip technology, this format is best used in a stationary position, as the disc player will 'skip' when jostled.

Although the CD player can be inexpensive by comparison to other technologies, the flip side is that CD audio books are the most expensive of the audio formats. Used audio books can be purchased at a reduced rate (plus shipping) from online booksellers. In the category of 'free is always better,' the library is the best source for CD audio books.

Portable Media Players (PMP)

PMP is an audio format associated with downloading music, but is also great for downloading audio books. Portable media players, commonly called MP3 players, are very small, palm-size and easily fit into a pants pocket. They have large storage capacities, allowing for hundreds of songs or books. Their popularity as a music downloading device, has decreased over the years as cell phones and tablets have the same capability for downloading music, videos, and audio books.

The functionality of PMPs varies from straight forward audio downloading technology to those that are able to download videos, movies, TV programs, and software applications, too. PMPs may have additional features such as built-in speakers, radio, camera, and recording capability. These units are understandably, more expensive. If you want a bare bones audio format for listening to books, there are some relatively inexpensive units that can be purchased.

Consider that there are other audio formats besides MP3, such as AAC, WMA, WAV, and Audible to name a few. If you intend to download books from one of the digital book stores, or your local library's website (Overdrive), make sure your PMP is compatible with their audio format. There should be a webpage listing compatible devices on those websites.

Look for Wi-Fi capability, otherwise a computer with internet connection is required to download to your PMP player.

The disadvantages, for the print disabled, is the small screens with teeny tiny print which makes it difficult to navigate through the menu choices. Speech output, such as Voiceover, which is available in the Apple iPod line of products, is very helpful. Within the audio text, there is limited capability to navigate forward and backward, not really knowing where you are going, until you get there.

Digital Accessible Information System (DAISY)

DAISY is an established worldwide standard for digitally produced reading material, whether it is books, textbooks, magazines, newspapers, or periodicals, that ensures material is accessible to all. It is a digital format standard for text and synchronized audio that can be accessed on various media players. The system is flexible enough to allow the print disabled to navigate through the audio text just as a sighted person can move back and forth though the chapters, subsections, paragraphs, or sentences of the reading material. Imagine a complete audio substitute for printed material. (8) Understandably, this has important implications for students and those in the work place who are print disabled.

The DAISY Consortium is a non-profit international organization that has set the standards. The guidelines are for a human sounding narration, synchronized time points in the audio to markings in the text, and navigation control. Within the standards, the amount of navigation capability may vary by the producer of the audio document (8) and the media player used.

There are three ways in which the DAISY file may be produced (9):

1. Audio Only. This DAISY format is most commonly used for recreational reading of books. The Talking Books of the National Library Service and Librivox are audio only DAISY-formatted books.

2. Text Only. These DAISY formatted documents will require a computer or digital reading machine that utilizes text-to- speech software. The quality of the narration is dependent on the software or device used. The Internet Archive and subscription services such as Bookshare (**bookshare.org**) utilize this DAISY format.

3. Audio and Text. The audio and text are synchronized. The user is able to follow along in the text while listening to the audio. This is helpful for the print disabled, because they can gather

information regarding the layout of the text such as paragraphs and sections, while listening.(9) The audio portion is read by a natural sounding voice. The subscription service, Learning Ally (**learningally.org**) provides audio-text synchronized DAISY formatted books.

Listening to DAISY

DAISY evolved as the switch was made from analog (remember the tape cassettes?) to digital in the 1990s.(10) It is not the only form of audio format. The DAISY formatted published information can be played on a variety of digital media players. That includes not only PCs and laptops, but reading machines (also discussed in 'Electronic Technology'), MP3 players, CD/DVD players, mobile technologies, such as smartphones and tablets, and a special category called the NLS Digital Talking Book Machines.

The flexibility to navigate will vary by the producer of the digital file and the media player. DAISY books are indexed or 'marked up' by the producer for ease of navigation. A novel will not have the same levels of navigation as a textbook will have. A novel may be marked up for the lowest level of navigation, such as, only by chapters. A textbook will be marked up at a higher level allowing for navigation, not only by chapter, but by subsection, page, paragraph, or sentence.

There are two ways to access DAISY audio and/or text:

1. Software application for computers and other mainstream mobile devices; and

2. Dedicated hardware called Digital Talking Book Readers.

Sources for DAISY books and documents are by way of internet download, CDs, SD (secure digital) memory card, or USB flash drive stick. The National Library Service (NLS) releases its books by way of a specialized, encrypted for copyright reasons Talking Book cartridge. Encrypted means the user must have an NLS encryption key to 'unlock' the book. The NLS will provide the encryption key to those qualified individuals to access encrypted DAISY books.(11)

Software for Digital Talking Books (DTB)

The software for reading DAISY formatted talking books can be downloaded from the internet or downloaded from a CD. The prices for the software applications are reasonable, that is, compared to text-to-speech software. There are also open source software downloads, meaning the software can be downloaded at no charge (**www.daisy.org/amis/download**). Minimum computer requirements are: speakers, a sound card, a keyboard, and a CD-ROM drive for those applications purchased on CD.

When making the software choice, consider these features: (12):

1. Operating System. It must be compatible with your system, either Windows, Mac, IOS, or Symbian.

2. Version and Type of DAISY Book Supported. Currently, most support DAISY versions 2.02 which is full text and full audio, and DAISY Version 3, which provides text and graphics only.

3. Audio Navigation. The program will guide the user through menus and options by a narrator's voice. No additional text-to-speech software required.

4. Capability to Highlight and Bookmark. The application highlights the text (when text is available) as it is read for those partially sighted who choose to follow along in the text. Bookmarking is for ease of navigation for future referencing.

5. Speed Reading. Need to get a lot of reading done? The software has the capability to speed up the narrators reading, without distorting the sound of the voice. This feature is very important for students and those in the workplace.

6. Languages. Some offer only one language (English), while others offer two or more languages.

Hardware: Digital Book Readers

These are the dedicated stand-alone digital readers. They range from small palm size units to larger, but still portable, table top units. There is a spectrum of units varying in capability. Some are simple readers designed principally to read books. On the other end of the spectrum are those with many features and applications designed as workhorse units for students and those in the workplace.

The features to consider when purchasing a Digital Book Reader are: (13):

1. Screen or No Screen. A few of the table top models have

screens. Similar to the computer screen monitor, it can give visual clues and will highlight text for the partially sighted. The smaller palm size readers, with a few exceptions, do not have a screen.

2. Control Panel. There should be controls for menu, power, play, volume, forward, backward, tone, and speed. Some units will have a full 12 number key pad with keys that serve double duty for navigating and accessing other features. They will also have large tactile buttons for reference, but only a few have large easy to read numbers and icons for low vision users.

3. Format Types. There is a wide range of text, audio, and DAISY (text and audio) formats. Familiarize yourself with the formats you will be using. A working individual may need to download HTML-formatted documents, while a student may need to download from **Bookshare.org** or Learning Ally, and a blind individual may desire to convert Braille files to audio. Keep in mind, not all DTB Readers have the capability to play the National Library Service Talking Book cartridges. This is a consideration if you are a qualified individual who is a serious reader who will buy a DTB because the Talking Book Reader provided by the cooperating library does not offer enough flexibility or portability for your needs.

4. Audio Navigation Cues. This is the voice that is activated as keys are touched. This is important for those with multiple keys with multiple functions.

5. Embedded Text-to-Speech Application. This opens up the option to have the digital text-only read aloud.

6. Types of Input Sources. Look for a headphone jack for private reading ability. USB ports are used to connect to PCs for downloading. These ports can also be used for attaching external CD drives, USB flash drives, and NLS Digital Talking Book cartridges, if compatible with the unit. SD memory cards can be used for storing data for later use.

7. Capability to Record. These units will have an internal microphone or port to attach an external microphone. Recording can range from recording short 'note-to-myself' messages to recording your own DAISY talking book and your own music. Although most have their own internal speakers and microphones, some will have jacks for external microphones and speakers.

8. Rechargeable Battery and Battery Life. Most all run on batteries that are rechargeable. Expect the unit to run for around 12 hours on a fully charged battery. Evaluate whether the batteries need to be removed to recharge, or are they recharged by plugging the unit into a plug-in wall adaptor.

Other bells and whistles include:

1. FM radio, clocks, and alarms are included with some units.

2. Voice recognition capability in which the DTB reader responds to basic verbal commands.

3. Wi-Fi capability so downloads can be made without having to attach to a computer.
4. Free manufacturer updates downloadable from their website.
5. OCR capability, so the unit can capture an image of text, say a menu or a form in a doctor's office. With the OCR activated, the DBT reader can read it to you.

A summary of available DTB readers and their features are available at: **www.daisy.org** >> Tools and Services >> Hardware Playback Tools, or check the following list of individual websites for a select number of readers.

Sources for Digital Talking Book Readers:

- **Bookport** by American Printing House for the **Blindshop.aph.org** >> Electronics >> Talking and Audible Products
- **Blaze EY** and **EZ** by HIMS **http://hims-inc.com/** Hims Inc. > Products > DAISY Players >> Blaze ET
- **Intel Reader** by Intel **www.intel.com/**
- **Milestone212 Ace** and **312** by Bones **www.bones-ch** >>products >> Milestone
- **Plextalk** by Freedom Scientific **www.freedomscientific.com** >>Blindness products >> Plextalk
- **Victor Reader Stream** by **Humanwarewww.humanware.com** >> on the go

Accessing the Digital World

There are many available online sources for e-books and audio books. Some will have monthly memberships with limits on the number of books downloaded. Other sellers charge on a per digital book basis. Audio books are always more expensive than e-text. There are several organizations that have made it their mission to preserve books in a digital format and have made them available to the world at no charge.

Textbooks Accessibility

Textbooks come in large print format, audio format, and also as digital text. PDF files, HTML, and other document formats can be downloaded, but be sure to check your e-reader manual to see what type of files can be accessed. Textbooks available for purchase as large print ,digital, and Braille, sources for text books are:

American Printing House for the Blind
1839 Frankfort Avenue
Louisville, KY 40206
800-223-1839
e-mail: **info@aph.org**
website: **www.aph.org**

Products: Books in large print, Braille, and digital audio format
for grades K-12.
Magazines in Braille and audio format.
Software for digital players,

Digital Players/Recorders.
Braille Products.
Products for Daily Living

Library Reproduction Service
14214 South Figueroa Street
Los Angeles, CA 90061
phone: 800-255-5002
website: **https://largeprintschoolbooks.com**

Products: large print school books, made to order. Any book can be made into a large print book.

Cost: per book basis

Digitally Formatted Textbooks:
Bookshare
480 California Avenue, Suite 201
Palo Alto, CA 94306-1609
website: **www.bookshare.org**
Non-profit source for books, textbooks, and newspapers. This source has text digital files (Daisy 3) for download to computers, mobile devices, or digital talking book readers with text-to-speech software. You must be a qualified registered member.
Learning Ally
20 Roszel Road
Princeton, NJ 08540
phone: 800-221-4792
website: **www.learningally.org**

Non-profit source for textbooks and literature in digital format, (Daisy 2.02 and 3). Must be a qualifying member and requires a membership fee. Grades K to college graduate.

Audio Books and More:

U.S. Library of Congress, National Library Service for the Blind and Physically Handicapped

The National Library Service is a federally-funded program to make books and magazines accessible (but not textbooks) to print disabled and those with physical disabilities that hinder their ability to read. Books and magazines are loaned out in Braille and recorded formats. Participation in this program requires that you are an U.S. citizen, and have documentation from a competent authority that you qualify. The qualified authorities are: professionals such as doctors, RNs, therapists, social workers, qualified educators, and hospital staff personnel.(14) The application form can be printed from the website. **[PDF]** Application for Free Library Service from the National Library Service.(15)

The program is administered by cooperating libraries. These are usually state, regional, or libraries designated as Braille, Talking Book, Blind, or Libraries for the Blind. There is a 'Find a Library' page at the website. Or call: 1-888-NLS-READ (1-888-657-7323).

Once your application is processed, the cooperating library in your region will send you a digital device. This Digital Talking Book Machine (DTBM) is a reader specific for the Talking Books format used by the NLS. There are two versions of the DTBM, which is lent to program participants. One is a very basic unit, while the other is a unit with advanced navigation for moving through text and bookmarking. You must specify which unit you prefer. Both are portable desktop units, with large tactile buttons.

The books come in the form of a digital cartridge. It looks like a cassette, but has a USB port. These cartridges will not be found or used in the general public. (16) That is how the NLS can make copyrighted literature available for free. This all arrives at your home (or institution) at no charge and postage is free. It is just as easy to return, again, postage free. (17)

NLS cooperating libraries will also have accessories like headphones, amplifiers, and pillow speakers. There are in the market place, available from accessibility technology developers, more advanced Talking Book digital devices with more features, like book marking, and greater navigating capabilities. (Discussed in the section: Hardware: Digital Book Readers.) Manufacturers of these devices will provide an NLS encryption key for those who qualify by NLS rules. (18)

A wide range of magazines are also available in this digital format to be read by the digital device. A participant can set up for an audio subscription. (19)

National Library Service and the Braille and Audio Reading Download (BARD)

For authorized users of the NLS service that have a computer and prefer to download digital talking books, the BARD system is available. You must first establish an account with the BARD system by application and create a user account name and password. Digital books are downloaded by way of the internet, from the NLS website to a computer. Then you transfer that file to a digital flash cartridge or USB flash 'thumb' drive. A blank customized NLS cartridge will need to be purchased. A list of those who sell cartridges is on the NLS website under Sources for Cartridges and Cables. This cartridge (or USB drive) can now be read on the Digital Talking Book Machine (DTBM).

BARD Mobile

Those who prefer the convenience of using their mobile devices, phone, tablet, or PMP, can download the BARD app. Interestingly, the on-screen controls look like the DTBM device. The app is supported on the iOS or Android operating systems. You must be a registered NLS user and have an account with BARD. The app is free, and can be downloaded from the app stores; iTunes and Google Play.

If you are interested in videos on how to use the BARD Mobile apps, type into your search engine bar: BARD Mobile "How-To" Series Webcasts. You can also search the NLS website for webcasts: www.loc.gov › Webcasts.

Music and The National Library Service

Music scores, books about music, and music publications can be accessed directly from the NLS in Braille and large print format. Audio formatted instructions on musical instrument playing and audio lectures and interviews are also available for the blind and visually impaired. Everything it seems for the blind or visually impaired musician, except for actual musical programs.(20)

Access for All:

The Gutenberg Project

This is a non-profit organization of volunteers that turns text in the public domain into digital format and makes it available to all by way of the internet. There are no fees or registration required to access these e-books.

The public domain means that those books are not under U.S. copyright, and most likely published before 1923.(21) Additionally, there are texts in which the copyright has expired, or been released by the owner of the copyright to Project Gutenberg.(22)

E-books can be downloaded directly from the site. The primary file format used is plain text, in that it has longevity and is an open format. When preparing to download, you will be given a choice. Most publications can be downloaded as free Kindle books. If you go to the Project Gutenberg website and search 'How to,' there is a very good section on how to get e-books downloaded to your device.

www.gutenberg.org/ >> Categories >> (H) How to >> (M) Mobile Reader Devices or (P) PDAs and ebook Readers

This is a good page for 'How to..' and app guides by device and operating system.

Project Gutenberg is partnered with **iBiblio** which is the public library of the internet. iBiblio is the website which lists collections of collections. They are also the main distribution site of the Project Gutenberg collection.

Visit: www.ibiblio.org/catalog/

Librivox

This is an affiliate organization to the Gutenberg Project, that provides books for free through the internet in digital audio format. Librivox is also run by volunteers who make public domain books available in audio format to the world. This website has a 'How to Listen' page that outlines several ways on how to listen to audio files. Visit: **https://librivox.org/** >>Help >> How to Listen

Other options include downloading by way of subscribing to iTunes through Librivox app, RSS feed, or accessing the files through the Internet Archive.

The Internet Archive and Open Library

The Internet Archive is an incredibly expansive source for not only books, but music, audio files, images, and video files. This too is a non-profit organization. All free, no membership required, and all through the internet. Visit: **www.archive.org/**

The Open Library is the internet 'catalog' of e-books. This is an online library book catalog, that is a porthole to other links. It is possible to download books to your computer, or help you to find a copy at another library to borrow or links to purchase books. This too, is a non-profit organization with a grant from the California State Library. Look under 'Help' to find tutorials on accessing e-books on Open Library.

For those patrons who are visually disabled, Open Library offers books in DAISY 3 text only format and encrypted DAISY format for use with the National Library Service Digital Talking Book (DTBM) reader. Encrypted means the user must have an NLS encryption key to 'unlock' the book. (23).

Your Local Library and Overdrive

If you are looking for more recent releases, the library, which is a good source of large print books and audio CD books, is also a good source for digitally formatted books and audio books to download to your PC, laptop, tablet, e-reader, or MP3 player.

Overdrive is the library e-book borrowing system, and internet access and a library card is all you need. Go to your local library website and look for the Overdrive icon or an option like 'downloadable media.' Overdrive is its own website, which has a library search site to find participating libraries should your local library not have downloadable books. On either site, you can find videos and instructions on how to use the service. Steps are given for downloading e-books and audio books to computers, e-readers by brand, and other digital media players. Look under 'Help".

Interestingly, your library will have a limited number of available copies, and you may find yourself "in-line" waiting for popular titles to become available. The amount of time you have for the loan is set by the library, and at the end of your time, you do not have to return it, because it magically expires. This means you do not have to make a conscience effort to return books. It also means a big surprise for procrastinators who may find that the book has disappeared from their e-reader. No late fees!

References

1. Large Print Weekly - HOME DELIVERY - The New York Times https://homedelivery.nytimes.com/.../LargeTypeWe...
2. Kitchel, J. Elaine, APH Guidelines for Print Document Design. American Print House for the Blind., www.aph.org/edresearch/lpguide.htm
3. NAVH Standards and Criteria for large Print Publications. www.sfgov2.org/ftp/uploadedfiles/mod/programmatic/NAVH06.pdf
4. eReader Screen Types. Retrieved from eReaderLookup.com
5. Offerstein, Tim. E-Reader Accessibility. IT Accessibility at Illinois, April 11, 2012, Retrieved from www.itaccessibility.illinois.edu/node/6
6. Top 10 eBook Readers of 2015. Retrieved from www.ebook-reader-review.toptenreviews.com/
7. Which Nook is Right for You? www.barnesandnoble.com/NOOK/U/compare-nooks/
8. DAISY Consortium, About Us. Retrieved from daisy.org >>about us
9. Kearney, Greg. DAISY: What Is It and Why Use It?, Braille Monitor, Feb. 2011.
10. DAISY/Print Disabled Books on Open Library (Open Library) FAQ, Retrieved from openlibrary.org/help/faq/accessing#read-a-daisy
11. DAISY Digital Talking Book. Introduction to DAISY, DAISYpedia. Hardware players. DAISY Consortium. Retrieved from daisy.org

12. Software Playback Tool.. DAISY Consortium. Retrieved from **daisy.org** >> Tools and Services >> Software Playback Tools

13. Hardware Playback. DAISY Consortium. Retrieved from **daisy.org** >>Tools and Services >> Hardware playback

14. **NLS: Sign Up for Service. - Library of Congress**. Retrieved from **www.loc.gov/nls**/ >> Home >> Sign up >> Eligibility for Service

15. **[PDF]Application for Free Library Service from the National Library Service**. Retrieved from **www.loc.gov/nls/pdf/application.pdf**

16. Frequently Asked Questions: Digital Talking Books. Retrieved from **www.loc.gov/nls/ Home >> About NLS >> digital books and Magazines >> Frequently asked questions: Digital Talking Books**

17. NLS That All May Read. Retrieved from: **http://www.loc.gov/nls/faq** Home >> Faq : Does it cost anything to use the program?

18. Sources for Cartridges and Cables. Retrieved from **www.loc.gov/nls/cartridges**/ Home > Sources for Cartridges and Cables.

19. NLS Reference Circulars. The Magazine Program of the National Library Service for the Blind and Physically Handicapped, NLS. Retrieved from **http://www.loc.gov/nls/reference/guides/magazines** Home > Reference > Circulars > Magazine Program.

20. Music Services What we can provide. Retrieved from **www.loc.gov/nls/**. Home >>What Services are Provided >>Music Services.

21. Copyright ,Public Domain, and Librivox (in the USA). Retrieved from **librivox.org/pages/public-domain/**

22. Copyright FAQ. Retrieved from **http://www.gutenberg.org/wiki/Gutenberg:Copyright_FAQ. All Categories >> (C) Copyright**

23. Learn about print disabled books on Open Library. Retrieved from **openlibrary.org**/ >>Help >> Learn about print disabled books on Open Library >> What are protected DAISY?

CHAPTER 18

Adaption Using Non-Optical Devices and Modifications for Activities of Daily Living

Adaption techniques discussed so far are optical devices (magnifiers and telescopes), electronic devices (video magnifiers and computer technologies), and visual adaptive techniques (eccentric fixation and scanning.) Although these devices and techniques can be used for many tasks, they are primarily geared toward reading the printed word. Literacy and the ability to see printed numbers and details are important for education, work, and activities of daily living.

Activities of daily living describes those activities we do outside of school and work. They are activities like watching television, food preparation, caring for personal needs, and leisure activities. Non-optical devices and modifications are compensatory techniques used to make life easier, safer, and more normal. There are several ways to adapt home life to accommodate your needs:

1. **Adapting the Environment;**
2. **Adapting Objects; and**
3. **Non-Optical Devices.**

Adapting the Environment

The extent in which adjustments need to be made to the living space for activities of daily living is dependent on the severity of the impairment. Someone who retains good peripheral vision and those who have mastered adaptive visual techniques, will not have the same concerns as those with more severe losses and have difficulty with orientation and mobility. Here are a few tips for a safe and accessible environment:

1. **Keep things familiar.** The furniture is best kept in locations that are easily maneuvered around. Small chairs and tables should be avoided, but if necessary, keep them in the same familiar location. Consider when purchasing new furniture their construction. Avoid chair and table feet and sharp corners that may be obstacles to trip over or cause bruising of the thighs.

2. **Maintain organization.** This actually goes along with keeping things familiar. Life becomes simpler if objects are in their place. Even those with good vision understand the frustration of tracking down misplaced keys, wallets, eyeglasses, etc. Have a place for everything and put everything in its place.

   Get rid of clutter. Lots of stuff on counters and drawers stuffed with bric-a-brac contributes to visual clutter and makes it difficult to find the more important useful items.

3. **Optimize the environment visually.** Start with lighting. Areas used for activities like food preparation, self-grooming, hobbies,

reading, and writing should have lighting that is bright enough and directed at the work surface. The kitchen table and counter areas should be well lit with overhead spot lighting and/or under cabinet lighting. Diffuse, center of the room lighting, is often not adequate. The reading and hobby areas should have adequate task lighting. For example, a 'gooseneck' flexible arm lamp can be placed over the shoulder to focus light to the work area.

Keep in mind that optimal lighting is an individual matter of preference. While most welcome the increase in light, others may be sensitive to higher light levels and will be bothered by the increase in glare. Experiment with different light bulbs and positioning of the light source. Also consider glare that might reflect off of glossy work surfaces. Use mats or darker surfaces to minimize glare. The optimal light level is the one in which you are comfortable and function the best without glare or loss of contrast.

Use color and contrast to highlight or outline objects within the environment. Optimizing contrast is maximizing the differences of reflected light off of objects and is manipulated by changing light levels or changes in color. Visually observing something with high contrast can make it more easily seen.

Stairs can be outlined with bright yellow 'caution tape,' which can be purchased in hardware stores. Bright, colorful broad 'duct tape' can be used to outline edges of tables, doors, drawers, light switches, or for labeling and organization. Many colorful duct tape options are available in the craft sections of stores along with colorful stickers, labels, and tags for high contrast and colorful visual cues.

4. **Make it your motto to "Be prepared."** Those with vision impairments don't like surprises. Be prepared for emergencies. Keep a well marked, easily accessible first aid kit in the house. Plug speed dial settings into the phone and clearly label emergency numbers. Even when out and about, make a mental note to know where the location of exits are. Think of it as being a secret agent in a movie thriller, always keep your senses attuned to your environment. Be aware of things like sounds and smells that other, normally sighted people might not notice. It is a skill you can teach yourself.

Adapting Objects

Within the environment there are objects that we use daily. Carefully select items that are user friendly. Adapting everyday items for ease of use can be done several ways:

1. **Optimize with color and contrast.** Look at table tops and counters. Select kitchen utensils or bathroom items that are brighter or that contrasts sharply against the flat surfaces.

2. **Choose bright solids over prints where possible**. A small object against a printed surface or container may not stand out, and get 'lost' in a decorative pattern.

3. **Organize and identify objects by labeling.** Organize items into groups that make sense to you. Keep certain cabinets and drawers dedicated to groups of items. Bins are also helpful for grouping like items on shelves.

   Color stickers, labels, tags, or bold markings in bold black or colored markers help identify objects. Use labels or markers to indicate frequently used settings on the dials of household appliances. The indelible marker, such as a Sharpie ®, comes in multiple colors and can be used to make broad visible markings.

   Adhesive dots, such as "Bump ons," are raised plastic dots that can be applied to frequently used settings on dials. Tactile writing pens, such as Hi-Marks®, are three dimensional plastic writing liquids in pen form, which can be used for labeling to make an object identifiable by touch. See the end of this chapter for sellers of these products. Dan Roberts, in his self-help guide, also recommends the puffy fabric paints found in craft stores, which can be used to give a 3-dimensional feel to labeling. (A Self-Help Guide to Non-Visual Skills by Dan Roberts. Distributed as a public service by Macular Degeneration Support, Inc. **www.mdsupport.org**.)

4. **Put household items to work for you.** Utilize the accessibility features available on your television and telephone services. See the section on communication and TV watching.

Non-Optical Devices

Specialty items can be purchased in department stores and online stores that make use of large print, larger size, or auditory feedback (talking devices) to adapt commonplace things that are used on a daily basis. Examples of items that are designed for those with impaired vision include:

1. **Large print and large size items.** There are many items made with extra large buttons and large print. These items can be found in department stores and in the mall. Commonly seen are big button phones, calculators, TV remotes, and pill organizers. Large print puzzle books, like crosswords, Sudoku, and word finders can be found in most book and magazine outlets. There are some more specialized items like large number scales, kitchen items with large markings and numbers, alarm clocks, and wrist watches that can be found only in specialty outlets.

2. **Items used to increase contrast.** Writing guides, also referred to as typoscopes, are black overlays used on paper. The black against white highlights the writing area. Bold, broad tipped pens contrast written words on white paper. High contrast bold lined paper can also aid the writing process.

3. **Devices that give auditory feedback**. These specialty items have a beep, tone , or talking voice that gives auditory cues. Watches, alarm clocks, and wall clocks can be set to give a tone at selected times, or have a voice that sounds out the hour. When taking care of personal business, talking calculators,

talking memo reminders, and taking caller ID makes it easier. Those with health concerns may find talking blood pressure and glucose monitors helpful. In the kitchen, there are even talking small appliances and cooking timers.

Talking labeling systems allow you to record descriptions of the labeled item. They utilize an electronic device, which when held near the special identification tag, recites a prerecorded description of the labeled item.

4. **Specialized magnifiers.** These are items with an attached utility magnifier for a specific task. Examples are magnifying tweezers, magnifying clippers, and syringe magnifiers. These items tend to be specialized and can be purchased thru low vision vendors. Magnifying mirrors for grooming are commonly found in department stores. In addition to magnifying, many mirrors have filtered light illumination.

Adapting to a Life with Low Vision: Putting It All Together

When reviewing this section, keep in mind that a few things need to be assumed. First, you should have received a comprehensive eye examination, and have eyewear that maximizes your residual vision. Second, there needs to be a desire and motivation on your part to accept the adaptions that need to be made in order to make it work. Finally, it can be difficult to make all the modifications on your own. Seek the help of an occupational therapist who is familiar with low vision rehabilitation and who can help you customize your life.

Writing

Writing is necessary for communication and personal finances. The handwriting of those with low vision can be notoriously bad. This is probably because details of the figures are not seen well enough. Taking your time and using your visual memory should help with having understandable handwriting.

Environmental Adaption. Adequate lighting and high contrast helps with writing.

Non-Optical Devices. Bold line paper, bold pens and felt tip markers contrast with white paper to aid in visualizing. Writing guides, which are usually black cardboard or plastic with cut-out rectangular slots, when overlaid on white paper give writing guidance where the contrast of the lines on paper, checks, and forms are not contrasted well enough to be seen. These guides are called typoscopes.

There is a writing guide specifically designed for check writing with the writing slots in the appropriate places for standard size checks. Large print checks and check registers can be ordered. Check with your bank to order.

Large button calculators with large print can be found almost anywhere and talking calculators are available through low vision vendors.

Optical Aids. These are optical magnifiers mounted on stands. They are raised above the paper and allow you to write beneath them.

Yellow lenses or filters help to decrease the glare off of white paper for those who are glare sensitive. They also increase the contrast of black and blue ink.

Electronic Devices. These are video magnifiers that come with a stand where you can angle a pen underneath to write. These typically have built in illumination. This is adequate for the short-term filling out of forms, writing checks, and short communications. If the need is for more extensive writing tasks, a CCTV has a larger field of view and does not require hunching over to see like you would with a smaller stand or video magnifier.

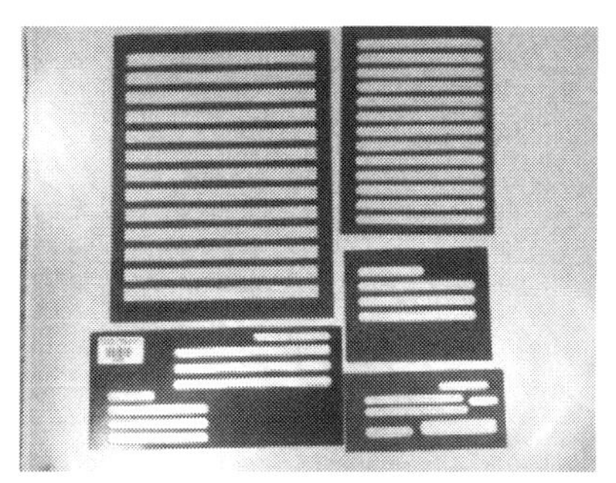

Typoscopes for high contrast

Communications

Specifically communications means telephones and telephone services. Check your telephone carrier's website for accessibility services.

Environmental Adaption. Contrast the telephone against the surface or wall where it is located. A white phone contrasts with dark counters or tables and vice versa,. black phones are best seen against white counters. This is especially advisable for the wireless phone. Who knows where the handset may end up!

Non-Optical Devices: Big button phones with large print numbers are commonly found either from a low vision specialty store, or through your telephone carrier. Select one that is user friendly, with the option to pre-set emergency and frequently used numbers. There are also large print and audible caller ID devices.

Your telephone or cable company will also provide large print bills if requested.

Object Adaption. Make use of telephone services. Check with your telephone carrier for the free information service: 411. This is a feature to help those who have difficulty reading the tiny print in phone books, which pretty much applies to everyone. The carrier will have documentation requirements as proof of need.

Label those preset phone numbers clearly and understandably. There are phones in which you can put a picture of the person associated with that number. This, of course, assumes that you can discriminate who is in that small picture. Consider labeling with colors, a couple of large letters, or use the tactile, colored plastic labeling pens.

Electronic Devices. Those who have adapted to the smartphone cannot live without it. The good news is that each manufacturer has a somewhat large screen version of their smartphone. Incorporated within the operating system are accessibility features for the visually and hearing impaired. Communication using tablets is possible by way of Face Time or Skype with other smartphones, tablets, or computers.

Watching Television

Environment Adaption. Get closer. This is the easiest form of magnification. Moving your chair from watching television at a distance of 8 feet up to 4 feet, doubles the size of the image.

Object Adaption. A big screen television is really nice.

Non-Optical Devices: Big button remote controls, with large print will help you easily surf the channels..

Optical Devices. Telescopes are used for viewing any distance beyond a meter (about 3 feet). Head-mounted binoculars are best used when sitting in a stationary position, like watching television. There are the off-the-shelf head-borne binoculars, and then there are the custom types which are measured and fit by your low vision specialist.

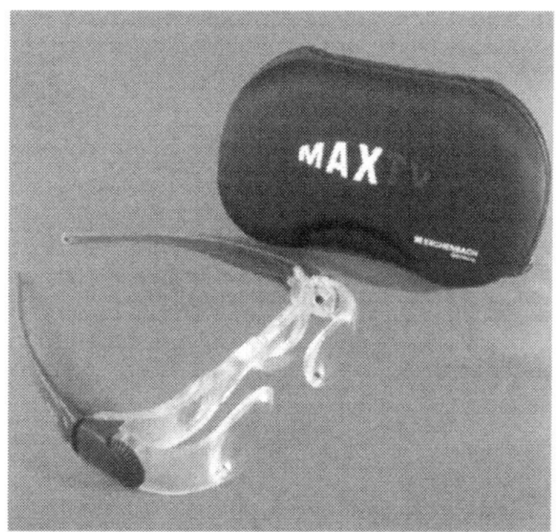

Photo: Binoculars for TV

Electronic Accessibility. Television accessibility is a work in progress. The Federal Communications Commission (FCC), has mandated that televisions made in the United States after December 20, 2016 must be accessible for the visually impaired. Those features which make television more accessible are:

1. Voice Guidance. This is a feature that when activated reads aloud the on-screen menu and any accompanying program descriptions. This feature can be either an option built into the television, or a premium feature offered by the cable provider.

2. Voice Commands. This is the ability to give verbal commands to control menu navigation and change channels. This is controlled through a voice-activated remote controller which has a microphone, and communicates with a smart TV. Check for this feature when purchasing a television, or through your cable/satellite provider and their own voice-activated remote.

3. Video Description (Audio Description). This is a pre-recorded audio description of the scene and action on the screen during pauses in dialogue. This is a product of the television network, and is available only for selected programs. When navigating through the menu, your cable company will indicate voice description with a symbol specific for voice description.

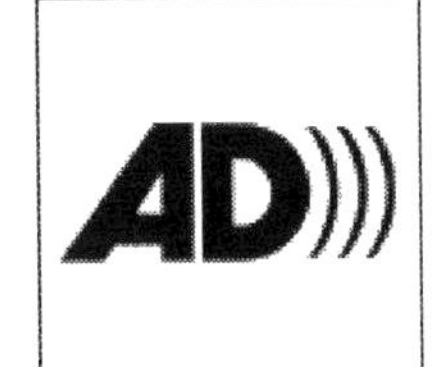

To determine if any of these features are available through your cable/satellite carrier, call or search for accessibility on the carrier's website. There should be a description on how to activate features using the remote.

Medical Needs

There are numerous devices that can be purchased for those who are independently caring for their medical needs, particularly for those who are diabetic.

Environmental Adaption. Organization is the key to keeping medications and supplies accessible. Devote a shelf or drawer to these items. Keep them in an order or groups that make sense.

Object Adaption. Ask your pharmacist for large print labels and large print medication information. The print size should be 18 point letter size. For reference, text of this book is 18 point.

As medications and supplies come in, label them in a way that is easy to remember and to prevent mistakes. If more than one of the same item is on the shelf, label by the date it came in, so the first item in is the first one used up. Use brightly colored labels with a large letter or pens that dispense three dimensional plastic for tactile clues for identification.

Non-Optical Devices: There are many, especially for diabetics:

- Weekly and monthly large print pill organizers. There are even some with talking timers and alarms as audio reminders;

- Talking thermometers;
- Talking blood pressure cuffs;
- Talking weight scale;
- Talking blood glucose meters;
- Large print syringes or syringe magnifiers;
- Adapters for medicine vials to center the needle; and
- Eye drop guides for dispensing eye drops.

Optical Devices. If it works for you, keep a magnifier handy in the area you keep your medications. Should there ever be any confusion, the magnifier would be readily available to give assistance. It doesn't need to be expensive, but it should help you see visual clues. Ask your low vision specialist or occupational therapist for recommendations.

Electronic Devices. There are talking medication bottles. It is a system in which the pharmacist is able to attach a special label to the bottom of the bottle. They can be used to identify the medication, dosage, and time to be taken. This label is read aloud by a bottle reader. The bottle reading device is loaned by the pharmacy to those who cannot read the medication labels. This talking medication bottle is not available at all pharmacies. Check with your pharmacist, mail order supplier, or Envision America (800-880-1180). Check the En-Vision America website, and click on the toolbar entitled 'Scrip Ability Find a Participating Pharmacy.' **https://www.envisionamerica.com/**

Personal Needs

Grooming and keeping personal items accessible makes life easier, and instills a sense of self-confidence and competence.

Environment Adaption. Get organized, both in the bathroom and in the closet. Clearly labeled bins on shelves or in drawers can keep those many small items that are stored in the bathroom organized, and prevents you having to buy more because you just can't find am item. Ladies, you know what I'm talking about! The same goes for sock and underwear drawers.

Remember to use lighting to help see into the closet. Stick-on battery operated lights can be purchased at hardware stores for dimly lit areas.

Non-Optical Devices. There are magnifying mirrors of various sizes, many of which are illuminated for personal grooming. There are also small tools like tweezers and clippers with attached magnifying lenses. (I have never had much luck with these.)

A few extra things for the visually impaired to consider are labeling tags for clothes hangers and sock organizers.

Electronic Devices. There are several talking electronic labeling systems which can be used to create descriptive labels for items in your closet and drawers.

A computer-type monitor with a mounted or free-standing camera can be used like a magnifying mirror, without the distortion. These units can be used for applying makeup, shaving, and grooming hair. The camera unit can also be manipulated to allow you to magnify other parts of your body, for example toenails, for grooming purposes.

Hobbies

Not all hobbies can be addressed here. These are just a few suggestions for visualizing details. Certainly, it will vary by the activity.

Environment Adaption. Good lighting with a well-placed task light is optimal. The work surface should contrast with the items you are working with and should not reflect light in a manner that causes glare off the surface.

Non-Optical Adaption. Figure out an organization scheme that makes sense to you and helps you to avoid the frustration of not being able to find pieces, parts, or tools. Holders, bins, and trays can be purchased at craft stores.

The easy thread needle is recommended for those that sew The opening is at the top of the needle, and you need only to pull the thread in a downward motion from the top. These can be purchased anywhere they sell sewing supplies.

Optical Devices. There are specialty optical magnifiers such as a neck borne hands-free magnifier, head-mounted magnifiers, loupes, and magnifiers that attach to sewing machines. There are also stand and hand-held magnifiers. The type and use of optical magnifiers is dependent on the activity. If you are confused by which device will help you, ask your low vision specialist or optometrist.

Photos:

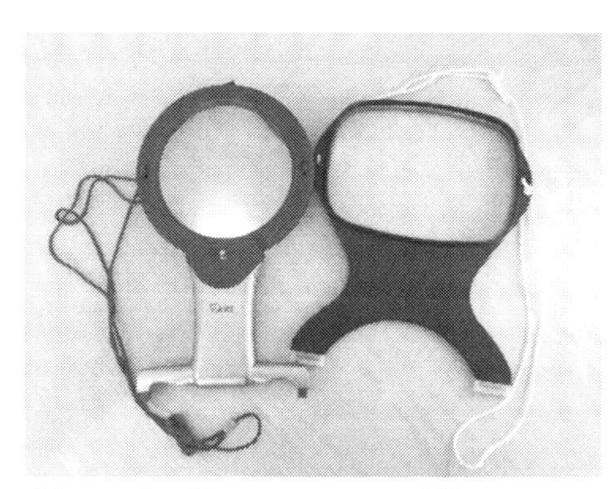

Hands free magnifiers

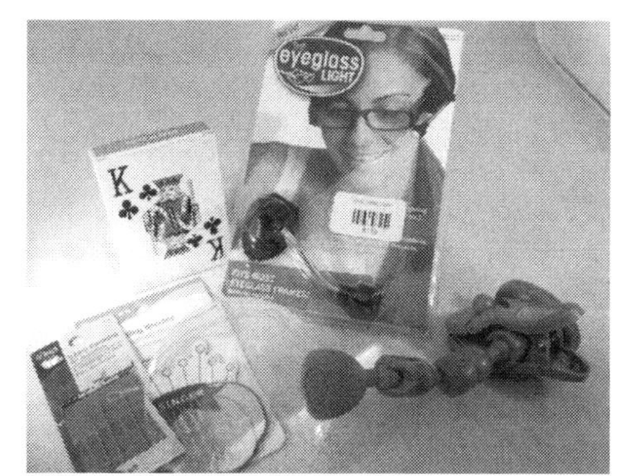

Easy thread needles, 'head light', specialty magnifier, and large print playing cards.

Electronic Devices. If working with small objects like coins or stamps, or assembling something where it is helpful to see the details, a CCTV is an ideal but expensive tool.

Food Preparation and the Kitchen

Environment Adaption. The work areas and counter tops should be well lit with lighting that is aimed downward at the surface. Under counter lighting works well, as does a light over the stovetop.

Optimize color and contrast. Use brightly colored or contrasting craft duct tape to give visual cues as to drawers, shelves, and switches.

Object Adaption. Organization and labeling can save time and aggravation when searching for products or cooking aids. Devote shelves and drawers for groups of utensils or products. Establish a system of organizing and labeling of products when they come into the house. Use those brightly colored labels with contrasting bold markings to label.

Cooking can be made easier by labeling frequently used settings on the stove, cook top, toaster, or microwave. Use indelible ink which is waterproof, tape labeled with a big arrow, the raised plastic ink pen, or stick on tactile dots, to label for tactile identification.

Non-Optical Devices: Large print cook books, measuring cups and spoons are designed not only for the visually impaired, but for those cooks who don't want to put their reading glasses on to cook. Utilize color contrasting with brightly colored measuring cups, measuring spoons, plates, glassware, and black and white cutting board options.

There are kitchen aids with large print digital readouts, and that give auditory feedback like microwaves, timers, cooking thermometers, and scales.

There are kitchen devices designed for safety: knives with guides, liquid level alerts, boiling alerts, and long oven mitts.

Optical Devices. Keep a hand-held magnifier in the drawer for instances where you need a little help with an appliance setting or small print on a packaging label.

Electronic Devices. Instead of a hand-held magnifier, a small or mid-size video magnifier is handy for occasional use. There is also a 'mouse-type' video magnifier, which when used in conjunction with a portable monitor, is handy for reading small print cook books and labels on cans.

Out and About, Shopping and Restaurants

While government buildings and medical offices tend to be more disabled accessible, restaurants and stores are not. Be prepared for the unexpected. It is helpful to stay with places you are familiar with, but that can be impractical and not as much fun. Grab your accessories and go. Here are a few suggestions.

Non-Optical Devices. Kudos to the U.S. government for changing paper currency to make it more easily identified and differentiated. Until the process is complete, the Bureau of Engraving and Printing is distributing, at no charge to qualified individuals, a currency identifier. For a limited time the iBill ® Talking BAnkNote Identifier, which is a small device you can attach to your keychain, is available. Go to the Bureau of Engraving and Printing website for the U.S. Currency Reader Program to download an application: **www.moneyfactory.gov/uscurrencyreaderpgm.html**..

Optical Devices. Hand-held spotting telescopes are useful for looking for signs and distant objects. Bioptic glasses are custom made glasses with a telescope mounted on or through the lens. These are most frequently used by those with low vision who drive. Because of the location of the telescope, which is mounted above the line of sight, it can be worn when walking around.

Small pocket size magnifiers are handy for checking prices or labeling on containers. Small pocket magnifiers that have a light are useful for reading menus in dimly lit restaurants.

Don't forget your sun wear as you step out the door. Even light tints with UV absorbing lenses provide protection on sunless days. Brimmed hats and visors give additional protection from stray light and glare.

Electronic Devices. Pocket size video magnifiers, which are illuminated by an LED light, are good for reading the labeling on products and reading menus in restaurants.

There are GPS devices designed specifically for the blind and visually impaired that gives step by step-by-step directions.

The smartphone surfaces again as a great accessibility device for shopping and getting around. There are numerous apps that can help provide GPS step-by-step directions, serve as magnifying tools, help read menus, and locate services. The key is to find helpful applications and learn to use them effectively.

The Bureau of Engraving and Printing has a U.S. Currency Reader App for the Apple iOS. EyeNote® is a free mobile app that uses the phone camera and the VoiceOver screen reader.

Recommended Reading

A Self-Help Guide to Non-Visual Skills, by Dan Roberts. Distributed as a public service by Macular Degeneration Support, Inc. **www.mdsupport.org**

Making Life More Livable: Simple Adaptions for Living at Home After Vision Loss. by Maureen Duffy, M.A., American Foundation for the Blind, 2002.

Navigating Life with Low Vision, Coping and Adjusting to Vision Loss by Tracy Stine. e-book. 2015.

Sellers of Low Vision Aids for Activities of Daily Living

Listed Alphabetically:

Assistech www.assistech.com/
4801 W Calle Don Miguel
Tucson, AZ 85757-1400 USA
Phone: 866-674-3549
International: +1-520-883-8600

Easily accessible website, multi-language.

The Chicago Lighthouse Tools for Living Retail
222 Waukegan Road
Glenview, Illinois 60025
Phone: 847-510-6200
http://chicagolighthouse.org/

Shop online or visit the store.

Independent Living Aids www.independentliving.com/
37 Ramo Street
Buffalo, NY 14207
Phone: 800-537-2118
Fax: 516-9373906

Free Catalog; call, apply online, or download.

Lighthouse Guild Store www.lighthouse.org
15 West 65th Street **info@lighthouseguild.org**
New York, NY 10023
Phone: 800-284-4422

Shop online or visit store.

LS & S Products www.lssproducts.com/
145 River Rock Dr.
Buffalo, NY 14207
Toll free, phone: (800) 468-4789
Fax: (877) 498-1482

Shop online or get a free catalog; call or apply online.

MaxiAids www.maxiaids.com/
42 Executive Blvd.
Farmingdale, NY 11735 USA
Sales Phone: 800-522-6294

Free catalog; order online a print catalog or a CDROM catalog

See bottom of the website to order a catalog for international language phone numbers.

CHAPTER 19

Low Vision and Driving

"Driving is a privilege, not a right." (Unknown)

"Privilege to drive," is an adage which describes the government perspective regarding the activity of driving. A privilege is granted and a privilege can be taken away. The 'privilege' to drive is an understandable philosophy if there are alternatives to driving. Instead of describing driving as a privilege or a right, necessity is a better term. It is a necessity for those who need to work and/or have no support system, and who don't qualify for government or other organizational assistance.

Not being able to drive can drop an otherwise independent, healthy adult into poverty, isolation, and despair.

This is not to say that every individual with little or no vision should have the privilege to drive. That would not make sense for safety reasons, not just for their lives, but for the lives and property of others. It is to say, that if an individual has reliable visual function, mental capability, and physical capability, they should be given the opportunity to prove themselves.

In regards to the right vs. privilege vs. necessity argument, review the Americans with Disabilities Act, Title II,

"…no qualified individual with a disability shall, on the basis of disability be excluded from participation in or be denied the benefits of the services, programs, or activities of a public entity, or be subjected to discrimination by any public entity."

Visual acuity is one factor of visual function, and visual function is just one aspect of driving.

Visual function encompasses several factors:

1. Visual Acuity. This is the easiest to measure and to attach a number. (Example: 20/20, 6/6, 0.0 log mar). It is the ability to see detail, and is the primary visual function cited for qualification for a driver's license.

2. Visual Field. This is another term for peripheral vision. It is a measure as to whether or not a person can see what is going on around them using their side vision. This is the other measure of visual function most frequently cited as a qualification for obtaining a driver's license. Although there are several ways to measure visual field, there is no standard testing method among departments of motor vehicles.

3. Color Vision. Red-green deficiencies are inherited, and can impact an individual's ability to accurately judge light signals. Color vision is often not tested, as deficiencies are not a criteria for denting individuals a driver's license.

4. Depth Perception. This is the ability to determine where objects are in the environment. An example is the ability to judge how far away your car is from the bumper in front of you. A person needs to have two functioning eyes to appreciate the highest level of depth perception. Although, there are monocular (only one eye) cues to depth, a person who recently has lost vision in one eye will have more difficulty picking up depth perception cues than someone who grew up with one functional eye.

5. Contrast Sensitivity. This is the ability to see a figure versus the background. Consider a dark grey car traveling toward you on dark grey pavement. The contrast for the grey car is lower than the contrast that a red car would have against the grey pavement. An example of someone with low contrast sensitivity is an individual with cataracts. Cataracts can create a haze and the environment will appear washed out or dull, and therefore will appear to have low contrast.

6. Glare Sensitivity and Recovery. Glare sensitivity means sensitivity to bright light and a slow glare recovery means having the slow ability to regain usable vision after exposure to a bright light. The significance is not just the annoying type of glare, but the debilitating type of glare. An example might be those on-coming halogen headlights or sun on the horizon which 'dazzles' and overwhelms your ability to see for brief or extended periods of time.

The act of driving is multifaceted. It is dynamic and requires the coordination of several human functions.

1. Vision. Previously discussed, is just one aspect.
2. Driving Intelligence. A successful driver knows the rules of the road. This is why the motor vehicle department gives a written test, but that is just the beginning. Driving involves lots of decision making, anticipation, and an understanding of traffic patterns, much of which comes with experience. However, driving intelligence is the ability of the individual to pay attention and learn the finer aspects of driving. (I believe there are a lot of people out there with driver's licenses that have really good vision, and little driving intelligence!)
3. Physical Ability. This is not just the ability to move arms and legs, as specialized equipment makes it possible for some disabled individuals to drive. It is also the ability to coordinate the activity of head, eye, foot, and hand movement in a timely fashion. Basically, reaction time matters, and the reaction needs to be an appropriate response.

So the question is: Should an individual who meets all the above mentioned physical and mental criteria, but is deficient, in part, to one of the vision requirements, be denied the privilege of a driver's license?

Legal to Drive

There is a great variability from state to state on regulations regarding driving privilege. Most states recognize that visual function is more than visual acuity, and have expanded the 'legal to drive' laws accordingly. State to state, the laws and regulations take a lot of twists and turns. Some are highly regulated and some are much more relaxed.

The Unrestricted License

What is most consistent between states are the requirements for the unrestricted license. Unrestricted licenses are issued to those individuals with a visual acuity of 20/40 or better in one eye (there are a few states which accept 20/50 and 20/60), and a horizontal visual field of anywhere from no requirements (not mentioned in the regulations) to 140 degrees. The horizontal visual field requirements are all over the place. There is almost every possible combination. Some states indicate binocular, while others reference monocular only. Some indicate both binocular and monocular. There are even states with vertical visual field requirements. All states allow monocular (one functional eye) driving.

The unrestricted license, allows driving anytime, anywhere. That is as close as it gets to uniformity.

The Restricted License

Most states issue restricted licenses for those with subnormal vision. It varies by state, but "restricted" usually refers to restricting things like time of day driving, distance, highway, and the use of vision accessories like the bioptic telescope.

Individual states require minimum visual acuity to be issued a restricted license. These minimums ranges anywhere from 20/40 up to 20/200. The Federal designation for 'legally blind' is 20/200. Some states require a special road test for the restricted license, while other states do not. The majority of states allow low vision drivers to use a bioptic telescope. There is variability as to whether or not the visual acuity through the telescope can be used to meet the minimum visual acuity requirements. Some states require training with the bioptic telescope.

Each state should have information online regarding state regulations for vision and driving. Some DMV regulations are easier to find than others. Your eye care practitioner should be able to provide information.

To find a summary of state licensing requirements in table format, see the American Automobile Association Exchange website (AAA): Drivers Licensing Policies and Practices Database, **http://lpp.seniordrivers.org/** .

Or search for your state's official vision standard. Type in the search bar: 'Your state' 'driver license vision standards.'

So the best guess answer to the question of vision and driving:

State regulations are designed for a margin of safety to protect the public, hence the designation of 'driving as a privilege.' What a search of literature has indicated is that much of the regulations and laws have no study or research basis as to the limits on visual function that determines at what level driving becomes unsafe.(1) Many have questioned: "how were these limits determined, by whom, and on what basis?" I could not find the answer, and apparently, looking at the wide range of state laws and regulations, neither could anyone else. Public officials have to set the line somewhere. As mentioned before, visual acuity is easy to measure and helps to establish a number for minimum standards. Other factors such as contrast sensitivity, glare sensitivity, depth perception, and night blindness are not so easily measured and quantified. Even visual field requirements have no standardized method of testing, and frequently are not tested by a state's motor vehicle department.

While some visual acuity requirements seem narrow, there is variability among drivers, some of whom may have other, not routinely measured, visual limitations that affects how they will function.(2) States legislate for what they can put a seemingly reasonable numbers on for public safety, without consideration of the individual's ability. That is to say, one individual with a VA of 20/100 vision may be a good driver, while someone else with 'better' 20/60 vision in combination with other visual, mental, or physical limitations may be a terrible driver.

The conclusion is that the privilege of driving is for those who meet the qualifications.(3) The low vision driver is limited by what can be measured, and from that, driving performance is assumed.(4,5) My theory is that experience is an important factor and low vision drivers are more attentive, drive more carefully, and take less risks.

Bioptic Telescopes

Bioptic telescopes are a driving accessory used by those with subnormal vision. A bioptic telescopic system consists of a miniature telescope mounted on a supporting eyeglass lens, commonly called a carrier lens. Most bioptic telescopic systems for driving have one telescope mounted through the carrier lens in a position just above the driver's line of sight. This mounted telescope is set at a slightly turned up angle of 10 degrees. Occasionally a bioptic system will have two telescopes (one for each eye). It is the single bioptic lens system that is used for driving.

There are two basic types of mountable telescopes. The smaller type is a Galilean telescope, which looks like a thick tube mounted through the carrier lens. The Galilean telescope is usually in the lower end of the telescope power range of 1.7X to 3X. The 'X' refers to 'times' magnification. E.g. 3X is three times larger than 1X magnification. The second type is the Keplerian telescope, which has the appearance of a bar mounted at the top of the eyeglass frame and lenses. This type allows for a more powerful magnification (4X and 6X). Because they are larger, they are also heavier. As with any magnifying system, the more powerful the imagination, the smaller the field of view. The smaller the field of view, the more difficult it is to localize an object of interest. The Keplerian telescope does have the advantage of a larger field of field of view in the higher powers vs. the Galilean in the same higher powers.

The bioptic telescopic system is used to enlarge the distance, so the details up the road can be seen by the low vision driver and therefore gives them better visual acuity. These devices can be used for those with subnormal central macular vision, but are not helpful for those with visual field loss.

The types of things a low vision driver may use the bioptic telescope for are signs, lights, traffic patterns further ahead, and roadside objects. Although detecting lights is not acuity dependant.. The bioptic telescope is not used constantly while driving, but is used intermittently and briefly to scan and spot. This is similar to how drivers use their side and rear view mirrors. Keep in mind; the peripheral (side) vision is just as important for monitoring surroundings and the flow of traffic, as it is most sensitive to movement. I am reminded of a horseback riding term called 'soft-eyes.' This is where the rider becomes acutely aware of the environment, utilizing all of their visual field and all their senses.

The eyeglasses that the bioptic telescope is mounted on will be the individual's regular prescription for seeing in the distance. That distance prescription would be for that person's optimal distance visual acuity, thus ensuring the best possible full field vision, which is what bioptic user relies on most of the time. If there is no prescription for seeing in the distance, the telescope will still need to be mounted in a set of non-prescription lenses as holders for the bioptic.

As mentioned before, the telescope is mounted above the line of sight and angles upward at a 10 degree angle. To spot an object, and get a better view of the detail of that object, the driver drops their chin slightly, causing the eyes to have to look up slightly. The telescope should be then precisely aligned, so that it is now level and the user is looking into the telescope straight ahead. The look is brief. The driver needs to be able to align and localize the point of interest in the telescope rapidly, and just as rapidly assess the visual information they viewed. The driver then quickly returns to full field viewing through the carrier lens portion of the bioptic telescope system. This takes practice, and a smooth riding car helps, as small head movements result in large sweeping movements when viewed through the telescope. The field of view through the bioptic is small (7 to 4 degrees) and the distant objects 'pop' into view. Lots of practice is needed to develop viewing accuracy.(6)

To learn more about the technique of using a bioptic telescopic system, take a look at:

- Coping with Vision Loss, by Bill Chapman, Ed.D, Hunter House Inc., Publishers, Review Section V. Pg 222 - 224.
- He describes his technique for scanning and spotting with a bioptic telescope.
- Chuck Huss, COMS, has a webinar on You Tube, in which he describes the training and skills needed to apply for a bioptic driving license. Type into the search bar: NOAH Webinar Recording – Bioptic Driving.

Properly fitted and aligned bioptic telescopes are not an off-the-shelf purchase. The bioptic lens fitting must be performed by a qualified professional, like an optician or optometrist, preferably by one who has done it before. These bioptic telescope systems can be very expensive. They are also not very attractive. The companies that mount the telescopes do not allow for thinner lighter fashion frames. The frame needs to be sturdy and are usually heavy plastic or heavy gauge metal. The carrier lens area does have to be large enough to allow for the mounting of the bioptic lens, and still have full field visibility.

Before you sign up for bioptic driving, check your state's regulations regarding the use of bioptics (39 states permit them at this time). While most states permit them, they may regulate how they are used in terms of strength of power, if they can be used to meet the vision requirements, and require special training programs. Your eye care professional will need to get involved. They can help determine if you are a candidate for bioptic driving. Once it is prescribed, you will need to be trained by a therapist to learn skills of scanning, localizing, and spotting. The next step will be to find a Certified Driving Rehabilitation Specialist. The specialist will train you to drive with your bioptic to meet the requirements of your state motor vehicle department.

Photos:

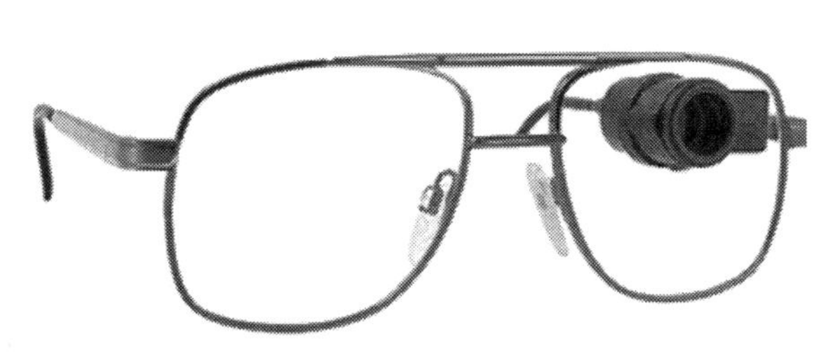

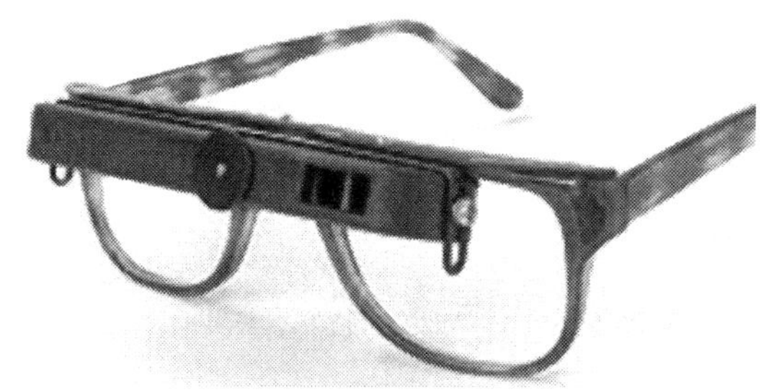

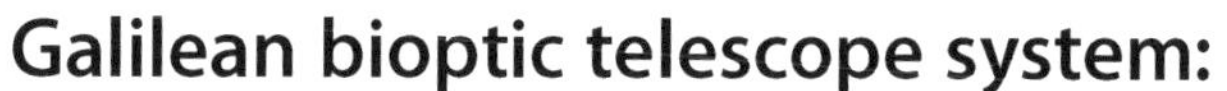

Galilean bioptic telescope system: **Keplerian Bioptic system.**

On a Safe Track

Safety is job number one. Here are some common sense tips to driving:

1. Optimize your vision;
2. Know your car;
3. Drive defensively;
4. Know your limitations; and
5. Drive legally.

Optimize Your Vision

1. A good set of eyeglasses with your best correction to maximize your visual acuity is the first step. A qualified eye care professional, who has worked with individuals with subnormal vision, will take the time to give you a good refraction for an optimal prescription.

2. Kick your eyeglasses up a notch with appropriate tints and anti-reflective coatings which can be added to that set of best corrected eyewear. (See Chapter 14 on Light, Lenses and the Eye).

   Tints are used to increase contrast and reduce the harsh glare from sunlight. The preferred tint for sunglasses for driving is a grey color. Grey tints are 'neutral' and do not change the color of signal lights. Yellow tints are good for increasing contrast, but a dark yellow or amber can impact your ability to identify signal light colors when driving.

Consider polarized lenses for sunglasses. Polarization reduces the reflected glare from flat surfaces like roads, water, and the hood and dashboard of the car.

Anti-reflective coatings applied to the surface of the lenses also reduces glare. A set of clear lenses with an anti-reflective coating is the best option for night driving. Your eye care professional can help with optimal tint selection and premium lens features selection.

3. Bioptic telescopic systems can be used by drivers in states that permit the use of these systems.

4. Consider installing a larger rear view mirrors which can increase the rear field of view. Panoramic mirrors are rear view mirrors that are larger, anywhere from 11 to 18 inches. Sellers claim they are easy to install, by fitting over your existing rear view mirror. This helps to expand the rear field of view to minimize the car's natural blind spots.

Know Your Car

1. Be very familiar with the dashboard and where all the controls are located. This is almost second nature if you have had the car for a while. What you don't want to do is try to read the numbers, or decipher icons, while driving. Once you start your car, before shifting into gear, check your gas gauge, set the temperature, check the mirrors, check the dashboard for warning lights, and

set the radio. There should be no excuses for fumbling around while driving.

2. Keep the windows and mirrors clean inside and out. A dirty windshield can be the source of glare, because incoming light is bouncing off the dirt on the windshield creating a veiling glare, making everything hazy. Visibility through a dirty windshield becomes most apparent when headed into the sunset or when diving at night.

3. Technology is your friend. If you haven't discovered it yet, global positioning satellite (GPS) devices are very handy to own. They can r help you anticipate turnoffs and lane changes; even if you know the route you are taking. The better GPS devices announce street names and route numbers, as this can also be very helpful.

Download a GPS app to your smartphone if one did not come preloaded. There are apps for speedometers designed for the purpose of displaying the speed numbers in a very large and visible format. In the App store, type in 'speed,' and select 'speedometer' on the dropdown menu. Car mounts for both smartphones and tablets can be purchased.

Another purchasable item, if your car does not already have it, is a parking sensor system. These systems give an audible signal of repeating tones to indicate your car is close to another object, and also has a digital readout for distance.

Some cars come with crash avoidance (prevention) systems, which have the ability to sense impending front end collisions.

These warning systems vary by their ability to auto-brake and stop or slow the vehicle.

If you have the opportunity to buy a car, check its visibility. Windows should be large enough to minimize those side and rear blind spots. Check the visibility though the front windshield. The angle of some windshields impart more glare off the dashboard than others. Look at the dashboard. Check to see that the gauge indicators are colored bright enough to see. Orange or white lines are easier to see than LED digital indicators for the print disabled.

We can all look forward to the day when cars drive themselves! (7)

Drive Defensively

This is a term coined by the National Safety Council that applies to everyone.

1. Don't follow too closely. Maintain the proper distance that will give you time to react and stop without incident. Remember from driver's education class, that distance is dependent on the speed of travel. The faster you are going, the further behind the other car you need to be.

2. Keep your eyes moving. Scanning your driving environment can give you the big picture and help you anticipate changes in traffic flow.

3. Anticipate the unexpected from the other drivers. Unlike the low vision driver, who is in high alert mode (right?!), other drivers may be distracted, or lacking the driver intelligence discussed previously.

4. Maintain a comfortable speed. Often other drivers may be driving faster than the posted speed limit. If someone behind you is pressuring you to go faster because they are in a hurry, well then, that other driver should have left earlier. If you are driving too slowly, however, that can be dangerous too. Comfortable to drive means you can keep pace with the rapidly changing demands of driving, in an appropriate and safe manner.

5. Telegraph to other drivers your intentions. Use your signals whenever appropriate. Also, let them know you are coming. Many cars have running lights that go on every time the car is started and are used even during the day.

Know Your Limitations

Avoid those situations that will shake your confidence as a low vision driver.

1. If reading signs is a problem, stick to regions where you are familiar with the streets and traffic patterns.

2. Avoid driving into the sunset (or sunrise) if you have a problem with light sensitivity or glare recovery. Headlights at night can also dazzle vision, making night driving difficult. If you must drive at night, as headlights approach, follow with your eyes the painted line on the right side of the lane that is opposite to the approaching car.

3. Choose the best times to drive. Driving east when the sun is rising, or west as the sun sets, can dazzle the vision of normally

sighted individuals and those with sub-normal vision alike. Avoiding bad weather conditions when driving is a good tip for all. Rain and fog and the dim light of an overcast day, combined with the glare of headlights can make visibility very difficult.

Driving at night is difficult because of the lack of visible detail, some loss of depth perception, and an overall decrease in visual field. Glare from oncoming headlights, contrasted with roads that are poorly lit and demarcated, makes it especially difficult for those with subnormal vision. These are the reasons why seniors quit driving at night as they get older, and why states restrict those with low vision from driving at night.

4. Stick to those roads less traveled if you become anxious in multilane traffic, stop and go roads, and large intersections. This can be done best by planning your route. Online map searches can give you a good visual idea of other routes to take. GPS devices provide alternate route instructions that you can select. It is better to check those out in advance.

Drive Legally

Know what your state's laws are regarding vision requirements for driving. Be prepared to take specialized training and testing.(3) Good chance it is going to cost you more to get your license than the average person. If it is determined that it is not safe for you to drive, know that it is for your safety.

Considering getting a drivers license? Here is a book for you:

- Driving with Confidence A Practical Guide to Driving with

Low vision. by Eli Peli and Doron Peli, World scientific Publishing Co. 2002 ISBN 9810247052.

For those young or newly visually disabled, who can't drive:

- Finding Wheels: A Curriculum for Non- Drivers with Vision Impairments for Gaining Control of Transportation Needs. Corn, Anne L., Rosenblum, I. Penny, 2000, ISBN: 9780890798270

Helpful websites:

To find a driving rehabilitation specialist in your area:

Association for Driver Rehabilitation Specialists, **www.driver-ed.org/** >> Directory & Services >>(dropdown)Member Directory and Search>> (click on)Driver Rehabilitation Specialist >>Select state on dropdown menu, click Search`

All about bioptic driving:

The Bioptic Driving Network www.biopticdriving.org. This website has additional information about driving, driver training, bioptics, and links to state driving regulations.

Driving with Low Vision at **VisionAware.** www.visionaware.org. >>Everyday living >>Transportation.

Bioptic Driving USA

Videos about Bioptic Driving:

YouTube:

Indiana Bioptic Driving Video by Bioptic Driving USA, Low Vision Centers of Indiana.

YouTube:
Type into the search bar: NOAH Webinar Recording – Bioptic Driving Chuck Huss, COMS

One Last Note:

Don't Let a Doctor Pronounce You Not Legal To Drive (or Legally Blind) Based on the Results of a Projection Chart Visual Acuity Test

Anyone who has had an eye examination is familiar with the chart projected on the wall that has the big E at the top. This is the customary Snellen chart. It has been around in different forms for over 100 years. Contemporary eye care providers utilize the Snellen chart mounted as a slide in a projector, which projects the letters on a screen. Sometimes the projected images bounce off a few other mirrors before it lands on the target screen. Testing a patient with this system is easy to control, flexible, and fast.

Even though it is the standard in eye care practices, the Snellen chart has its flaws. Most who use the Snellen chart know this, and for most of their normally sighted patients, it is not an issue. It has variability in the legibility of the letters, letter size, and the distance between letters and lines of letters. There are a different number of letters per line. This means that if you were to miss two letters on the 20/80 line, it is certainly more noteworthy than if you were to miss two letters on the 20/30 line. There is also variability between manufacturers of Snellen charts and projector systems. Not all projectors are created equal. There can be variability in projected light and contrast.

It is significant to potential drivers, that there are no lines of letters between 20/100 and 20/200. If your vision is 20/125 and your state allows for a restricted license, but no license is given to those with 20/200, testing with a Snellen chart is a problem for you.

Those researchers who need to have quantifiable and accurate visual acuity measurements for research and treatment of ocular disease will use what is called the ETDRS chart. Although there are many other charts, this particular chart was developed for the Early Treatment Diabetic Retinopathy Study (hence ETDRS). The letter sizes and legibility are equal, spacing is calculated proportional to letter sizes, and there are the same number of letters per line. This chart also has two lines of letters between 20/100 and 20/200. So it is possible to test for the in-between acuities of 20/125 and 20/160. This ETDRS chart bypasses the pitfalls of the projection chart. The letters are high contrast black on a white opaque plastic which is back illuminated in a 'light box.' The lighting is consistent and the contrast is high. This is what the FDA considers the gold standard for research for accuracy and reproducibility.

Is your doctor guilty of malpractice because he does not use the ETDRS chart? Absolutely not. The Snellen chart works well for the vast majority of normally sighted patients. As flexible, easy and fast as the projection system is, the ETDRS chart system is slow and it is more difficult to test patients. These more specialized charts are found at referral centers and where research and clinical trials are being done.

There have been several studies completed that compare the Snellen and ETDRS charts, predominantly for the assessment of the results of research and clinical trials. The studies found no significant difference in measured visual acuity for those patients with normal or near normal vision. (8) However, those patients with moderate vision (worse than 20/40) and those with severe loss of vision (worse than 20/200,) did notably better with the ETDRS chart than with the Snellen projection chart measurements. The improvement was as much as 2 lines better with the ETDRS chart. (9, 10) This means that a patient whose visual acuity is 20/200 (legally blind) with the Snellen chart, you could conceivably be measured at a better acuity of 20/125 with the ETDRS chart. Those who should expect to do better with the higher contrast, better illuminated ETDRS chart are those who have higher contrast and luminance needs.(9)

If you are borderline between legally blind or are borderline for a restricted license, it might be worth your while to request a referral to retest your visual acuity at an office or a center that has an ETDRS chart.

Photos:

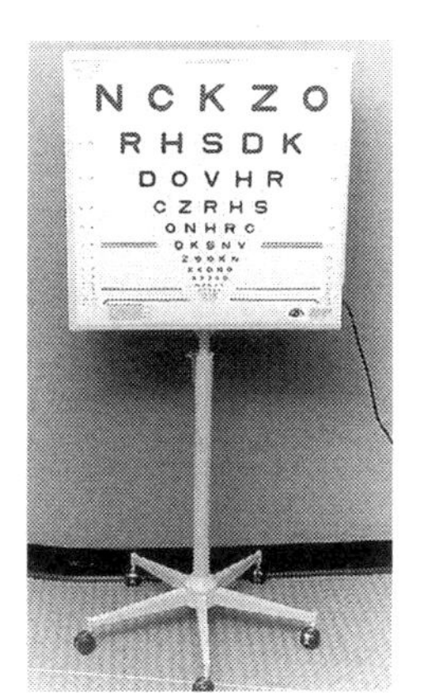

ETDRS chart

Snellen projection chart

References

1. Peli, Eli. Driving with Low Vision: Who, Where, When, and Why : Retrieved from **www.serinet.meei.hardvard.edu/faculty/peli/papers/Ch401-y0016pdf**.
2. PDF: Vision Requirements for Driving Safety. International Council of Ophth., Dec. 2005, Retrieved from **www.icoph.org.pdf**.
3. Peli, Eli, Peli, Doron, Driving With Confidence A practical Guide to Driving with Low Vision, World Scientific Co.Pte.Ltd.,2002.
4. Chapman, Bill. Vision and Driving A Literature Review and Commentary, Ophthalmic Physiol Opt. 1997 Sep;17(5):371-91.
5. Owsley, C., McGwin, G. Jr. Vision Impairment and Driving, Surv. Of Oph.,1997, 43: 535-550.
6. Chapman, Bill, Coping with Vision Loss, Hunter House Publishers, 2001, section, Chapter 34, pg 222.
7. Rosenthal, Dr. Bruce P., Kelly, Kate. Living Well with Macular Degeneration Practical Tips and Essential Information. New American Library, 2001, Chapter 12 pg 193-193.
8. Kalpan S., Kartnick J., Jayaajini S., Comparison of Static Visual Acuity between Snellen and Early Treatment Diabetic Retinopathy Study Charts, International Journal of Educational Research and Development. Vol.2(3), pp 82-88, March 2013. Retrieved from: **http://www.academeresearchjournals.org**.
9. Falkenstein, Iryna A., et al. Comparison of Visual Acuity in Macular Degeneration Patients Measured with Snellen and Early Treatment Diabetic Retinopathy Study Charts. Ophthalmology. Feb. 2008, 115(2):319-323 Retrieved from **www.ncbi.nlm.nih.gov**.
10. Kaiser, Peter K., MD, Prospective Evaluation of Visual Acuity Assessment: A Comparison of Snellen versus ETDRS Charts in Clinical Practice (An AOS Thesis). Transactions of the American Ophthmological Society, 2009 December, 107:311-324. Retrieved from http:// **www.ncbi.nlm.nih.gov**

Appendix

Visual Acuity Notation, Conversion Table

Metric	Snellan	MAR	Log MAR	Decimal
6/60	20/200	10	1.0	0.10
6/48	20/160	8.0	0.9	0.13
6/38	20/125	6.3	0.8	0.16
6./30	20/100	5.0	0.7	0.20
6/24	20/80	4.0	0.6	0.25
6/19	20/60	3.2	0.5	0.32
6/15	20/50	2.5	0.4	0.40
6/12	20/40	2.0	0.3	0.50
6/9	20/30	1.6	0.2	0.63
6/7.5	20/25	1.25	0.1	0.80
6/6	20/20	1.0	0.0	1.00

Amsler Grid

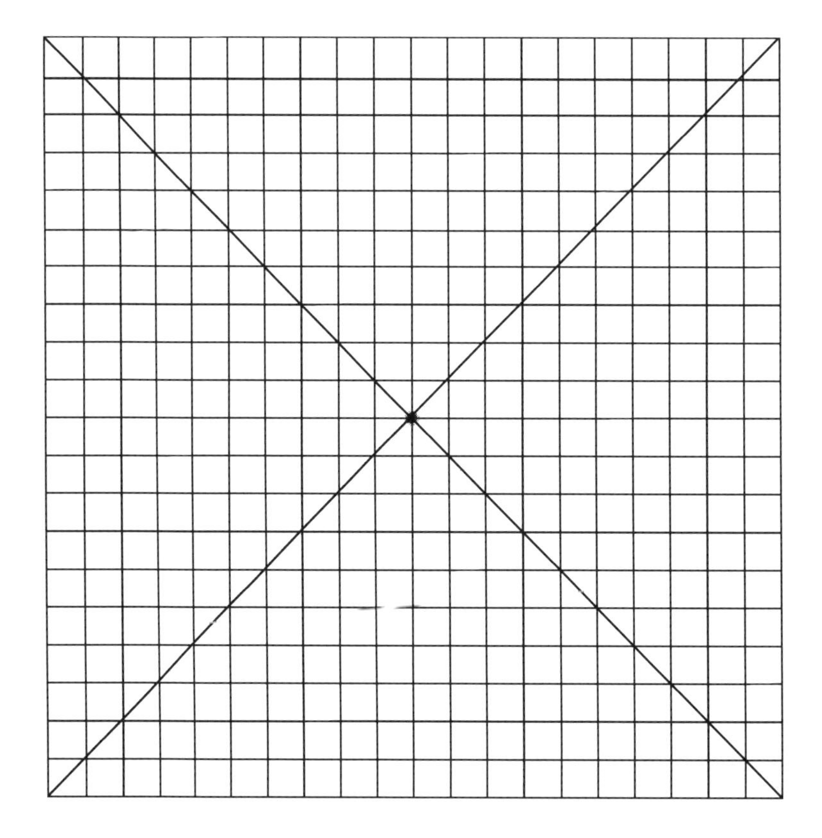

Cover one eye. Hold the chart 28 - 30 cm from your uncovered eye. This book is nearly 28 cm in length (11 inches).

Keep your eye focused on the center of the chart, and observe:

- Can you see all four corners and sides ?
- Are there any places where the lines of the grid are missing or blurred?
- Are there any places where the lines and squares are not straight?

Computer Font and Visual Acuity Chart

Life is good.	72 pt		
Good things will	48 pt	20/400	8M
come to those who	36 pt	20/320	6.3M
wait. That is what they say.	28 pt	20/250	5M
But don't wait too long, as	26 pt		
life may pass you by.	24 pt	20/200	4M
Live like there is no	22 pt		
tomorrow. Cherish	20 pt	20/160	3.2M
each day as it comes.	18 pt		
Believe that if you ask	16 pt	20/125	2.5M
you will receive. Life is	14 pt		
good and good things	12 pt	20/100	2M
will come to you.	11 pt		
Life may not be easy.	10 pt	20/80	1.6M
It is how we accept the challenge	9 pt	20/63	1.25M
that makes the difference.	8 pt	20/50	1M

Hold at 16 inches (40 cm).

Bibliography

Brown Barbara. The Low Vision Handbook for Eyecare Professionals. Second Edition. SLACK Incorporated, 2007.

Chapman, Bill, Ed.D., Coping With Vision Loss, Maximizing What You Can See and Do. Hunters House Publishers. 2001.

Corn, Anne L., Koenig, Alan J., Ed., Foundations of Low Vision: Clinical and Functional Perspectives. AFB Press, American Foundation for the Blind, 11 Penn Plaza, New York, NY, 1996.

Crandell, John M., Jr. PhD., Robinson, Lee W., EdD. Living with Low Vision and Blindness. Springfield, Illinois, U.S.A., charles C. Thomas, Publisher LTD. 2007.

Dickinson, Christine, Low Vision Principles and Practice. Oxford, Auckland, Boston, Johannesburg, Melbourne, New Delhi, Butterworth - Heinemann, 2002.

Faye, Eleanor E., M.D. Clinical Low Vision. 2nd Edition. Boston/Toronto, Little, Brown, and Company, 1984.

Faye, Eleanor E.,MD, Albert, Darren Lee, MD, Freed, Benjamin, OD, Seidman, Karen R., MPA, Fischer, Michael, OD. The Lighthouse Ophthalmology Resident Training Manual. A New Look at Vision Care. Lighthouse International, 2000.

Freeman, Paul B., Jose, Randall T., The Art and Practice of Low Vision. 2nd Edition. Boston, Oxford, Johannesburg, Melbourne, New Delhi, Singapore. Butterworth-Heinemann, 1997.

Hall Lueck, Amanda, Ed., Functional Vision, A practical Guide to Evaluation and Intervention. AFB Press American Foundation for the Blind, 11 Penn Plaza, Suite 300, New York, NY, 2004.

Jose, Randall T. Editor, Understanding Low Vision. AFB press, American Foundation for the Blind, New York, 1989.

Langdell, Cheri Colby, PhD, Langdell, Tim, PhD. Coping With Vision Loss, Understanding the Psychological, Social, and Spiritual Effects. Santa Barbara, California, Denver, Colorado, Oxford, England. Praeger, 2011.

Merin Saul. Inherited Eye Diseases, Diagnosis and Management, Second Edition. Boca Raton, London, New York, Singapore. Taylor & Francis Group, 2005.

Moses, Robert a., Hart, William M., ED. Adler's Physiology of the Eye Clinical Application. 8th Edition, St. Louis, Washington, D.C., Toronto, The C.W. Mosby Company, 1987.

Nowakowski, Rodney W., Primary Low Vision Care. Norwalk Connecticut, Appleton & Lange, 1994.

Peli, Eli, Peli, Doron. Driving with Confidence A Practical Guide to Driving with Low Vision. New Jersey, London, Singapore, Hong Kong. World Scientific Publishing Co. Pte. Ltd.,2002.

Rosenthal, Bruce P., kelly, Kate. Living Well with Macular Degeneration, Practical Tips and Essential Information. New American Library, 2001.

Scheiman, Mitchell, Scheiman, Maxine, Whittaker, Stephen G., Low Rehabilitation, A Practical Guide for Occupational Therapists. SLCAK Incorporated, 2007.

Index

A

F

G

H

I

J

K

L

M

N

O

P

R

S

T

U

V

W

X

Made in the USA
Monee, IL
30 May 2020